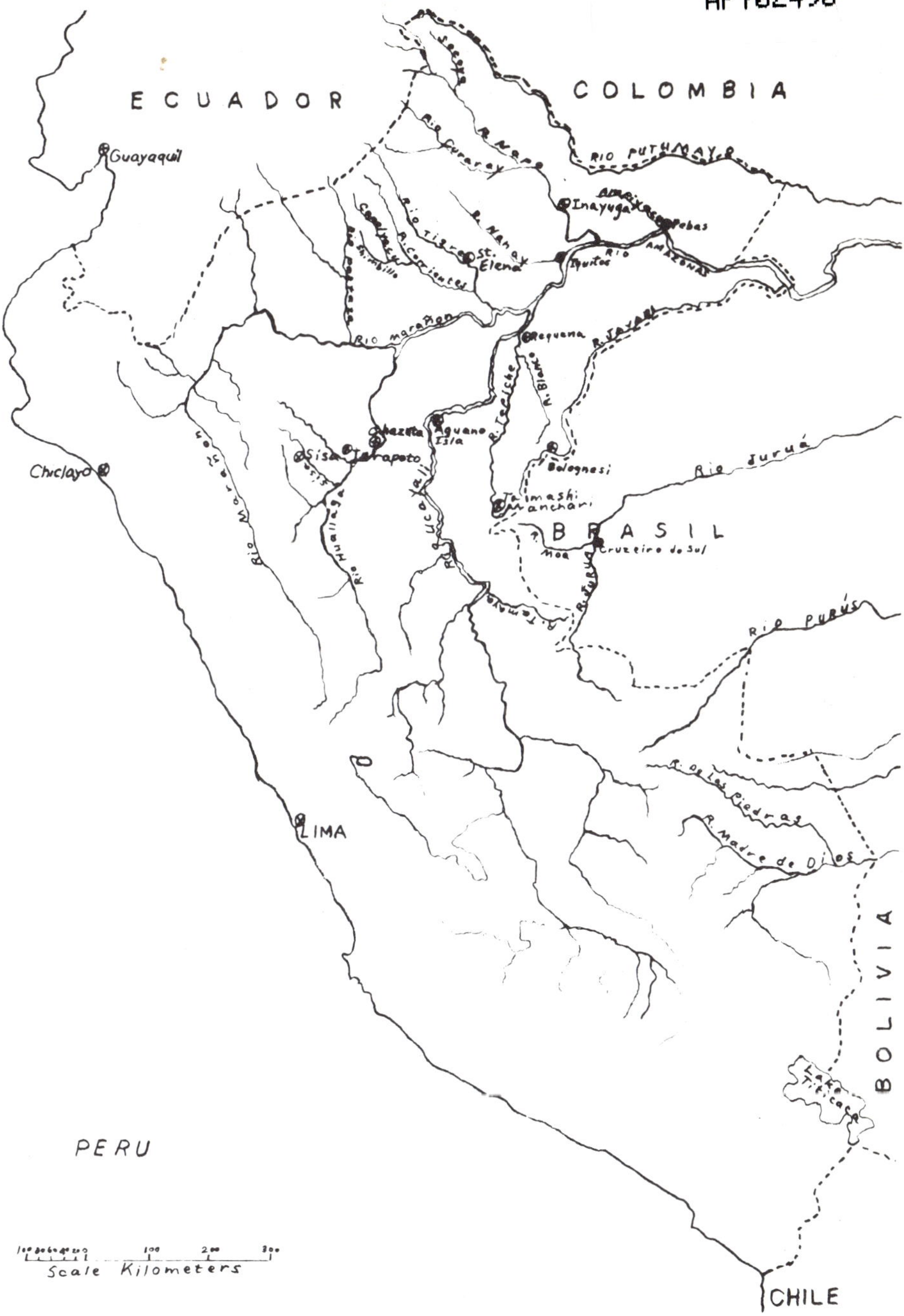
ECUADOR
COLOMBIA
Guayaquil
RIO PUTUMAYO
Rio Curaray
R. Napo
Inayuga
Pebas
Iquitos
Rio AMAZONAS
St. Elena
R. Nanay
Rio Tigre
R. Corrientes
Rio marañon
Requena
R. JAVARI
R. Blanco
Aguano
Isla
Tarapoto
Sisa
Chiclayo
Bolognesi
Rio Juruá
BRASIL
Moa
Cruzeiro do Sul
Rio Huallaga
Rio Marañon
Rio PURUS
R. de Las Piedras
R. Madre de Dios
LIMA
Lake Titicaca
BOLIVIA
PERU
Scale Kilometers
CHILE

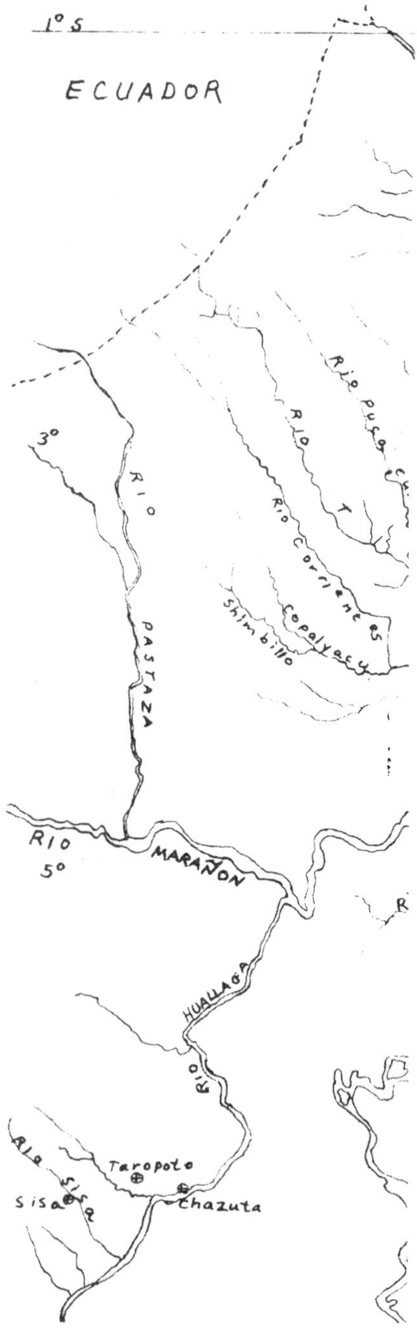
1° S
ECUADOR
3°
RIO
PASTAZA
Rio Corrientes
Copalyacu
Shimbillo
RIO
5°
MARAÑON
HUALLAGA
RIO
Taropoto
Chazuta
Sisa
Rio Sisa

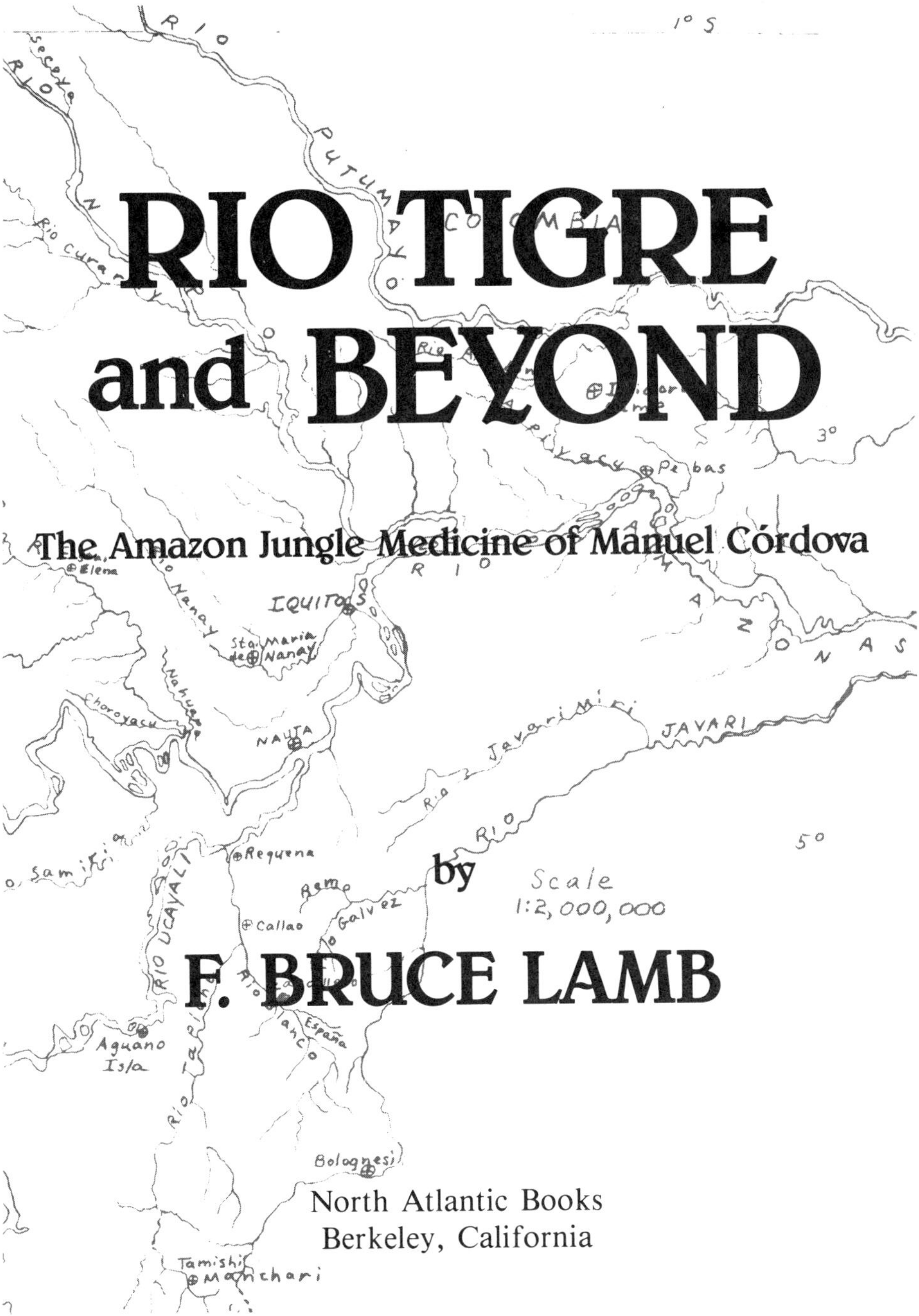

RIO TIGRE and BEYOND

The Amazon Jungle Medicine of Manuel Córdova

by

F. BRUCE LAMB

North Atlantic Books
Berkeley, California

Rio Tigre and Beyond
The Amazon Jungle Medicine of Manuel Córdova

ISBN 0-938190-59-8 (pbk.)
ISBN 0-938190-60-X (cloth)

Publisher's Address:
North Atlantic Books
2800 Woolsey Street
Berkeley, California 94705

Cover and book design by Paula Morrison
Typeset in English Times by Classic Typography

Rio Tigre and Beyond is sponsored by the Society for the Study of Native Arts and Sciences, a nonprofit educational corporation whose goals are to develop an ecological and crosscultural perspective linking various scientific, social, and artistic fields; to nurture a holistic view of arts, sciences, humanities, and healing; and to publish and distribute literature on the relationship of mind, body, and nature.

Library of Congress Cataloging in Publication Data

Lamb, F. Bruce (Frank Bruce), 1913-
Rio Tigre and beyond.

Bibliography: p.
Includes index.
1. Córdova-Ríos, Manuel, 1887- . 2. Amahuaca Indians—Medicine. 3. Medicine-man—Biography. 4. Indians of South America—Peru—Medicine. 5. Ayahuasca. I. Title.
F3430.1.A5C625 1985 615.8'82'0985 85-11429
ISBN 0-938190-61-X
ISBN 0-938190-59-8 (pbk.)

For Carolyn

who has been deeper into these
esoteric modes of consciousness
than most of us

Acknowledgements

I wish to acknowledge the inspiration of the late Professor Harley H. Bartlett of the Department of Botany, University of Michigan, for arousing my interest in the tropical forest environment and for the suggestion that local informants in the tropical milieu (even if uneducated from our standards of judgment) could make an important contribution to a newcomer's understanding of how complex tropical forest ecosystems operate. In addition I want to acknowledge the following people who contributed directly to the development of the manuscript: Dorothy and Maurice Kamen-Kaye of Cambridge, Massachusetts for a critical appraisal of an early version of the work; Kenneth and Johnnie Baker of Iquitos, Peru, and Orangeburg, South Carolina, for their hospitality during work on the manuscript and for encouragement during the process of its creation; Rafael Pereira of Lima, Peru, for advice and assistance during a critical series of background interviews with Manuel Córdova at Lima, Peru; Allen MacKenzie of Ardsley, New York; William J. Higginson of Paterson, New Jersey; Manuel Escudero of Topeka, Kansas, for critical reviews and helpful suggestions on improvement of the presentation of the story; Willard Johnson of Vista, California for finding a home for the manuscript; and to my wife Elizabeth for assistance in bringing the manuscript through its various transformations. My special thanks go to Richard Grossinger for editorial effort beyond the call of duty.

Contents

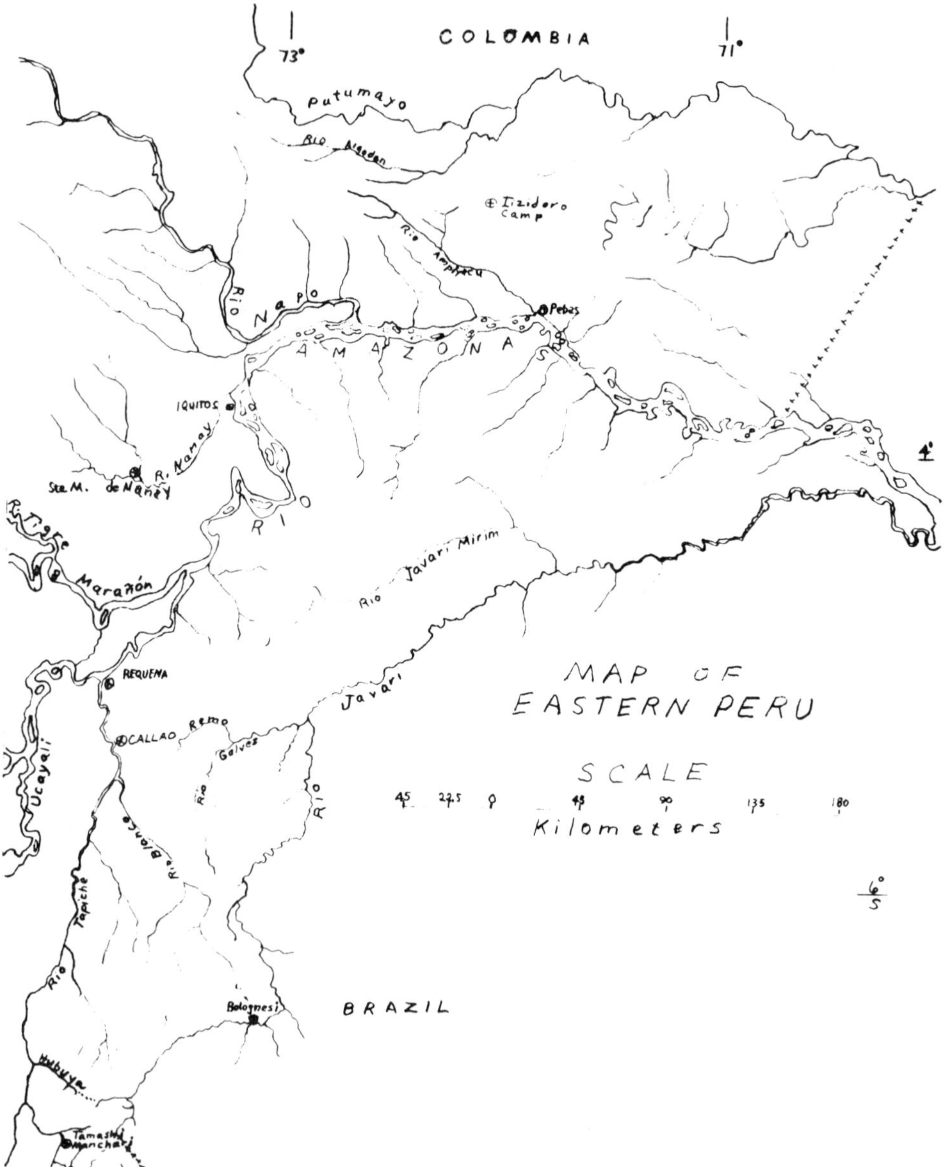

COLOMBIA
73°
71°
Putumayo
Rio Algodon
Izidoro Camp
Rio Ampiyacu
Rio Napo
Pebas
AMAZONAS
IQUITOS
R. Nanay
Ste M. de Nanay
RIO
R. Tigre
Marañón
Rio Javari Mirim
4°
REQUENA
Javari
MAP OF EASTERN PERU
SCALE
45 22.5 0 45 90 135 180
Kilometers
CALLAO
Remo
Galves
Rio Blanco
Rio
Ucayali
Rio Tapiche
6° S
Bolognesi
BRAZIL
Hubuya
Tamashi mancha

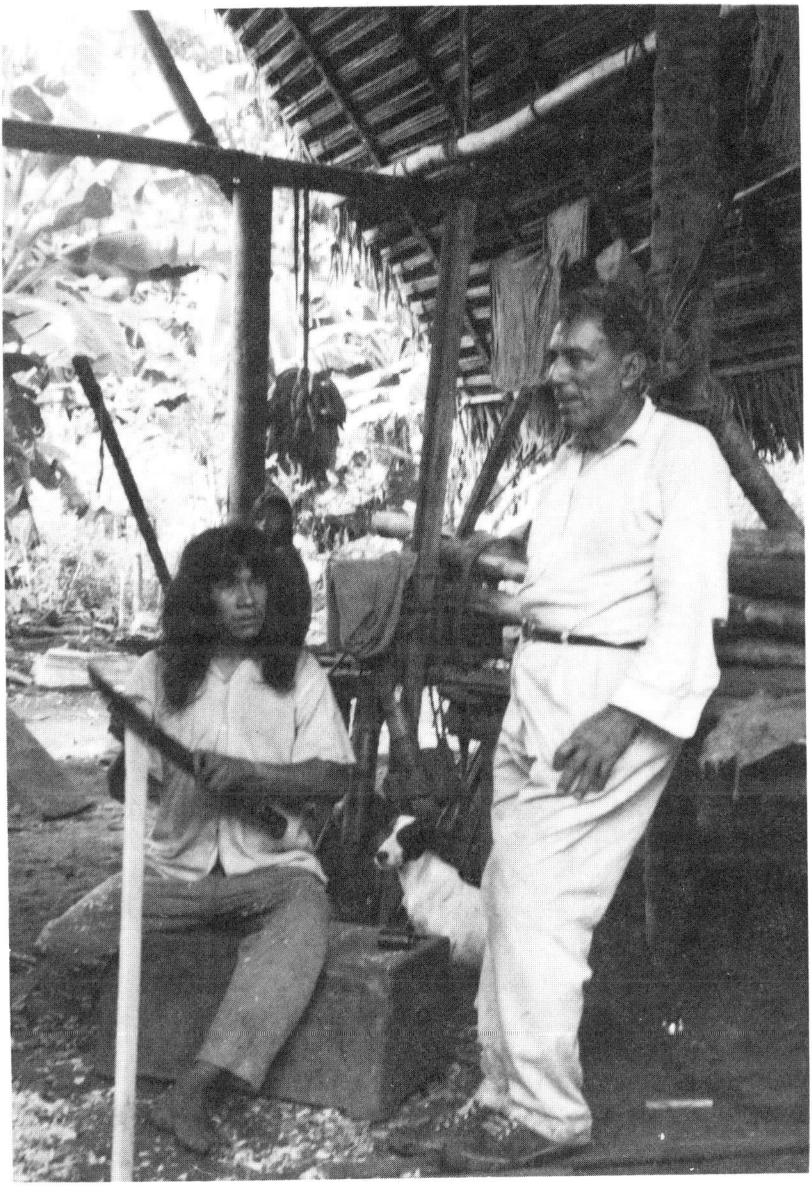

Manuel Córdova with Murato Indian shaman on Rio Shimbillo tributary of Rio Tigre, Peru 1961

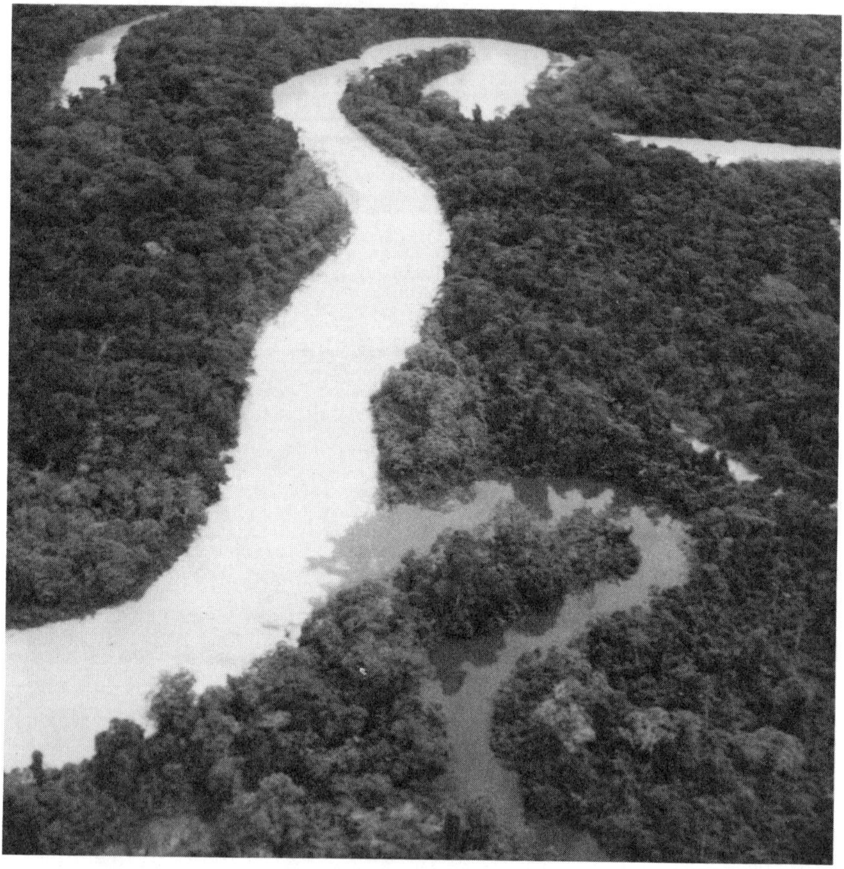

Meandering upper Amazon tributaries. *Photo by F. Bruce Lamb*

Preface
The Most Curious Beasts in the Forest

> "Since man is a product of nature, I believe that a cure for all of his ills will be found in nature and these cures are natural, in my opinion, and not miraculous at all. But that is part of another story."
>
> Manuel Córdova, in *Wizard of the Upper Amazon*[1]

Fulfilling Manuel Cordova's promise of another story, F. Bruce Lamb's *Rio Tigre and Beyond* recounts an unparalleled Amazonian adventure, completing the life story of Manuel Córdova Rios who at the very beginning of this century was abducted by Native American tribals to be trained as their new shaman. Here he remembers the rest of his life, a series of missions and adventures guided by his pre-Columbian training but in the context of the upper Amazonian Peruvian river city of Iquitos, in a world intricately changed by its millennial contact with the imported Columbian civilization. If we are fascinated by the elusive archaic world of our common human heritage, it is because we are so isolated from it, ignorant of its knowledge and its mysteries. Intolerable is life divorced from these our most ancestral voices, for now we have discovered, as civilization, since Columbus, has reached into the last pockets of surviving prehistoric peoples, that only a few individuals in this century have crossed the line dividing us from that other originary world to know something of the experience of the first peoples.[2]

The world in which we live today began in 1492 when Columbus linked the Old to the New World. Within a few centuries no point on the globe had been untouched by the pan-global Columbian exchange. Only in a few remote areas did the pre-Columbian world survive the mercantile nineteenth century—in those parts of the earth so far away as not to be worth finding or exploiting until rubber cutters, responding to a new demand for raw material in the early 1900's, opened the heart of the jungle forests of the Peruvian headwaters of the Amazon River, disrupting the life and territory of native clans. To provide new leadership, the old chief Xumu captured and trained one of these young Peruvian rubber workers as his replacement, so for seven years in the first decade of this century Manuel Córdova lived in as pre-Columbian a world as has survived on this earth in recent times.

While a forester in the upper Amazon in the 1960's, Bruce Lamb was entrusted by Córdova with the story of those seven years, subsequently publishing the book *Wizard of the Upper Amazon* in England and the United States.[3] This *Rio Tigre* book begins with a summary of that account and I too will draw from it because these two books, this and the *Wizard*, must be read now as one. Had not Lamb returned after that publication to Peru in 1972 to record more remembrances, we would not have this complete life sequence, but he sought Córdova out over a period of four more years, on and off during visits, to bring the life to its maturity and through its later episodes. Córdova was born in Iquitos on November 22, 1887 and died there on his ninety-first birthday in 1978.

These chapters constitute a remarkable memoir. However, do not expect an autobiography, or a systematic ethnography. These remembrances focus on episodes and meanings, going in circles, as shamanic inspiration does. Lamb did not approach Córdova to record and collect systematic data, as that almost surely would have shut him up forever. So these are analects, the rememberings of a lifetime. Anecdotal and self-revelatory, this book is thereby ever more precious an account, for it tells the story from the inside, not from the outside as we would have to do. No wonder we come away from Córdova's life memories stunned emotionally and challenged intellectually, or mystified and skeptical.

Now that both parts of Córdova's life story can be united into one life image we can begin to understand the significance of his initiation into the knowledge ways of a pre-Columbian Native American peoples. Without this second book we have no way of assessing the significance of the jungle Indians' way of knowledge which felt Castanedesque or fantastical. As the final pages of the *Wizard* book ran out, unanswered questions arose. What happened after Córdova's return to Iquitos? What was the manner of his life, after seven years in pre-Columbian Amazonia? Did he use the archaic knowledge he learned and for what vocation? These are vital questions since only with their answers, contained in this book, can we make any sense, ultimately, or give any evaluation of Córdova's transformation in an apprenticeship to a primeval science from a stratum of human evolution prior to our own.[4]

To recapitulate briefly, in the *Wizard* book Córdova recalled his seven years in the pre-Columbian world. In a shamanistic initiatory transformation the old chief Xumu directed the young Córdova through an apprenticeship which gave him knowledge of nature, as much as our physical sciences seek, but through different means. Here we have a chance to compare our means of knowledge with those of aboriginal times as they were taught to Córdova. He was trained to be the specialist in ecstatic knowledge, the role typical of the shaman (sometimes called the "chief" or the "medical person"). First, they ritually incorporated the kidnapped teen-ager into the social fabric of the tribe. Then, after six months, the chief led him into a deliberate course of initiatory transformation, beginning with restrictive diets, herbal purges, baths, and massages, and culminating in a series of vision experiences using their native ecstaticant, *ayahuasca*. In the first experience, Córdova underwent ecstatic transformation, initiated by a violent shock to the nervous system, and in the second, a violent muscle spasm followed by a release into ecstatic ways of knowing, dream-like visionary states no longer limited by conscious identification with the physical body (having the "impression of being free of my body, capable of actions, sensations and knowledge completely divorced from my physical being." *Wizard,* p. 37).

Córdova noticed after these first two initiations into the ecstatic knowing state that he was changing in his ordinary life too, learning the native language and identifying more with his Indian captors in their common environment. He found them extraordinarily well adapted to their home forest. From the wizard chief's ways he saw how the state brought on by the vision vine was used to gain knowledge concerning the empirical world in whatever way was needed, such as to help hunters increase their success in securing game or to improve the culture's social integration. Then in a series of remarkable teaching visions Córdova's mentor instructed him telepathically in the indigenous tribal lore and its special access to reality, thus both passing his power on and instructing him in the knowledge he would need to be the new chief. Córdova acquired shamanic powers, knowledge of plants as food and medicine, and developed psi powers,[5] including precognition, locating objects at a distance, and knowing how to help and handle others for their own well being. When the old chief finally died Córdova filled his new role and expanded his knowledge and powers in renewed vision sessions, until, after seven years, he escaped to return to his home far from the pre-Columbian jungle. Upon reentry he had to accustom himself again to wearing clothes and was so dismayed by his first expedition through the streets of Manaus that he was left utterly at a loss.

Though young, Córdova had done two nearly impossible things: He had survived, not as a slave but as a pre-Columbian shaman, and then he made it back to his own world again. In that other world, did Córdova's experiences bear any relationship to ours? Or was this passage, beyond the Columbian exchange, into the world before ours just a sleepwalk through fantasy realms we in rightful wisdom have long ago left as superstition and falsehood? The noted Harvard Museum Botanist Richard Evans Schultes remarked in his review of the first edition of the *Wizard* book, "Many experiences and happenings in the story might strain the credulity of all who have not lived themselves amongst Indians in primitive Amazon societies."[6] Indeed this proviso leaves most of us predisposed to skepticism, and thus liable to miss something important. We should not dismiss the account so easily, however, as our current cultural predispositions lead us to do. Nor should our evaluation hang on the use of the ecstaticant *ayahuasca*, since it worked merely as the active placebo which initiated and trained Córdova in ecstatic knowledge, an effect which can be produced with appropriate expectation by a thousand different triggers including sound, ritual, meditation and sensory deprivation.

What strikes us about this account in the *Wizard* is precisely its genuineness. Here is an account, finally, from the inside, of an apprenticeship to shamanic knowledge and power in a setting uncontaminated by the Columbian culture. The chief's initiatory training led Córdova to extrasensory wisdom, releasing mental powers and accessing valid knowledge of the physical realm of reality in which survival goals succeed or fail. This archaic knowledge depended on ecstatic aquisition and transmittal which is the shamanic equivalent of our writing systems, schools, libraries and elaborate techniques to store, retrieve and transfer information. Nature was the object of this special esoteric path, so Córdova's medical science rests on a thoroughgoing naturalism, quite in contrast to the supernaturalism characteristic of later agricultural and urban peoples. To be the group's shaman, Córdova was taught a special psychic way of knowing, and he acquired the culture's accumulated tradition, especially medical knowledge. He thus received a pre-Columbian initiation into that epistemology and medical paradigm, as uninfluenced as any we have come upon by Columbian reality.

To have this second part of Córdova's reminiscences is treasure indeed. Now we can ponder the meaning of this life transformed by pre-Columbian knowledge.[7] Most meaningfully, he became, in his mature years, a master healer. This did not happen all at once. Though Córdova was fully possessed of knowledge by his early twenties when he returned to Iquitos, his healing career did not become central to his life until the later years of his third decade, after marriage and occupational farming. As he remembers it, he first used his knowledge of the jungle to explore for timber or to discover and extract *curare* or rubber. These are wonderful episodes when Córdova returned to the native world. Then, once he began married life, he was called on to use his medical knowledge to help his family and workers, and, ultimately, people who came to him, recommended as he was with each success. By 1929, just beginning his forties, he settled in Iquitos where he spent the remaining fifty years of his life devoted to worldly pursuits, including a cock fighting ring, while continuing to serve his patients. Implicit in true knowledge and initiation is the commitment to others. Manuel Córdova's life, as we see it in these pages, so humbly remembered, exemplifies a human commitment, a way of life which uses knowledge for others.

One model of human maturation we can identify from shamanistic times is that of ecstatic initiation, for those specially chosen by constitution or vision, and a life spent using the special access to ecstatic or psi knowledge for the service of others. This was the model of Córdova's life. As he remarked to Lamb: "I could never turn suffering people away when I had it in my power to help. . . ."

We have in this work a priceless record of a genuine Native American medicine, something like a light in near void of reliable information about the pre-Columbian world. Unlike most travellers behind that curtain of irreversible time who do not become incorporated into the other world, Córdova was taken completely over. His record provides us with extraordinary material on the medical knowledge of nonliterate peoples, which almost always has been fragmentary, based on outside or secondary sources, or, worse, on careless accounts of casual observers. Our lines to prehistoric reality have long been compromised by a complex of various world-view and reality-paradigm biases held by various observers and investigators, missionaries, explorers, exploiters, military and merchant visitors and anthropologists. Their cumulative bias hampers our attempts to describe or interpret archaic medicine, which is easily dismissed as being more magical than medical. Such reasoning concludes that anything which does not fit into our current scientific paradigm necessarily is magic (i.e., entirely fantastic). The medicine of Manuel Córdova was not magic or supernaturalism but a naturalism, like those of early Greece, and of all Sino-Siberian-influenced cultures, including both of the Americas, as well as science itself. This book allows us to confirm that preliterate medical traditions treated disease as effectively as our scientific medicine, something Córdova demonstrated countless times in his doctoring, often as the last resort of patients given up by Western scientific doctors or poisoned by their treatment.

Córdova comments on our medicine in these pages, speaking skeptically of our medical categories and treatment strategies, our potent drug substances and the cold rationalism of our care of patients. He looks at our medical practice from the perspective of an holistic naturalism akin to Chinese and Native American holism. He thinks our doctors do not bother to understand the real underlying problems of their patients which create their symptoms and diseases, and thus they have a medicine for everything but a cure for nothing. He repeatedly received patients poisoned and devastated by excessive drug usage (as when antibiotic treatment caused an asthmatic condition which he corrected using the extracted juice of a certain large forest snail). Synthetic antibiotics and food substances, he observes, stay in the body, toxifying it, so that any attempt to get at the underlying bodily malfunction will necessarily require preliminary detoxification. Some of these medicines create cancer-like conditions largely iatrogenic in origin.

Córdova was a true bi-cultural healer. Profoundly influenced by and trained in a pre-Columbian world, a founding member of an upper Amazon Masonic Lodge, he also acquired technical medical knowledge from Western-trained doctors through his Masonic connections. Able to make direct comparisons between his multicultural multitemporal healing model and that of Western medicine, Córdova regularly finds his own to be more precise and superior.[8]

Córdova's healing art involved several skills characteristic of shamanistic specialists around the globe. First, he used a visionary psi state to gauge the nature of problems, whether medical or other. Specifically, *ayahuasca* provided Córdova a visualized access to the bodily systems of his patients to make shamanic psychic diagnoses. Córdova used *ayahuasca* as a diagnostic and prognostic vine, but not as a healer. As Córdova says, "*Ayahuasca*, it tells you how, but by itself it cures nothing directly." Notably, in later years he no longer needed to use the vine. Rather he entered the psi-diagnostic state "by uninterrupted contemplation of the subject alone at night." In this state he visualized the body's various systems until he identified the trouble.

Secondly, he would psychically visualize the specific natural remedy for the pathology. He also gave inner attention to adequate preparation of the patient, and the technicalities of extraction and dosage. Further, he carefully observed the patient's progress and responses to his remedies, occasionally even taking the diagnostic vine potion to examine and correct his procedures.

Unless we admit that in a clairvoyant psi state one human being can see into another person's body to assess the blood system or identify a black malfunctioning liver, or unless we consider it possible that correct plants can appear in prognostic vision, along with exactly how to prepare and use them, we will fail to understand Córdova's medicine. It is not miraculous but as natural and as cognizant of physical reality as ours is. Córdova's ancient science forces us to make such an admission. He directed his cures through a part of the mind most of our current psychologies have not even mapped yet, the whole realm of psi having only recently come to the attention of our researchers.

Córdova's psychic healing arts were complemented by a strong sense of patient phenomenology, so a third component of a healing course was to include patients psychologically in the cure. If they believed in witchcraft and evil spirits, they would have to be convinced as part of the cure that they had been exorcised. Córdova healed by combining natural treatment and wise observation of the patient, uniting body and mind. However, he had little good opinion of those who make a show of healing while failing to back it up with adequate specifics at the bodily level.

What we are immediately inclined to discredit in the healing career of Manuel Córdova, either by reducing it to magic or aggrandizing it to the level of the miraculous, turns out to be quite reasonable and human. It is archaic, yes, but valid in its veridical reach into physical reality, and a part of human knowledge which we have learned for generations to consider untrustworthy. What a fate our oldest traditions should suffer at the hands of our reluctant self-understanding! Córdova's life above all demonstrates that already in prehistory human beings had the fullest human understanding of maturity and deliberately could direct some persons in ways of growth to bring them to the most useful and noble human knowledge. His life as a doctor indicates that pre-Columbian ways can be of immeasurable value to modern people.

It is interesting that at the very same time Bruce Lamb was taking down the adventures recorded in the *Wizard* book, a young anthropologist, Marlene Dobkin de Rios, took up residence not far away from Córdova's home. She lived in Belem, an urban slum of Iquitos precisely to study *ayahuasca* healers, resulting in her book-long study, *Visionary Vine,*[9] followed by a diverse set of articles[10] on disease conceptions and healing practices of these *maestro curandero-ayahuasqueros* in Iquitos. One of these, "The Vidente Phenomenon in Third World Traditional Healing: An Amazonian Example,[11]" provides information on don Hilde, a *vidente* or medical seer from the nearby river city of Pucallpa, Peru. Her book on don Hilde will be invaluable because like this one it will provide detailed biographical material on the life and practice of an *ayahuasca* healer. As a result of the pioneering work of Lamb and de Rios, others now have made this phenomenon the object of scholarly research. The articles of Luis Eduardo Luna document later developments in Iquitos.[12] Also around the same time that Lamb and de Rios gathered their early materials, the anthropologist Irwin Press christened the phenomenon "The Urban Curandero" in an *American Anthropologist* article.[13] What we have in this book then is an example of Latin American urban *curanderismo*, part of an acculturative adoption of native Amazonian medicine[14] by the new residents of Latin American urban centers.

A cursory review of this literature, however, bequeathes us yet another dilemma of interpretation: Though these observers have identified and described urban *curandero-ayahuasqueros*, none of them really resemble Manuel Córdova beyond certain technical similarities, such as using the vision vine or having recourse to traditional herbs.[15] Apart from these traits, rather obvious dissimilarities distinguish how Córdova practiced with the diagnostic vine from the treatments of these other practitioners. Differences in etiology and ascribed function are obvious. Rather than looking psychically into the body of the patient, *they* look for etiologies in the practice of witchcraft and evil spirits, with treatment requiring in most cases an exorcism (which Córdova did only when the belief system of his patient required it). Often in the case of the other *ayahuasqueros* they would give the vision vine to patients in group healings, something Córdova never mentions doing; rather, in his case, it was to aid him to access psychically relevant body systems for diagnosis, then to visualize herbs and regimens of treatment.

Perhaps the urban context introduces so many new factors into human life that renewed etiologies and therapies arise to cope with greater psychological complexity, and the psyche itself becomes an object of treatment, along with or rather than the body. Córdova worked at the mental level but he mobilized the forces and balances of the bodily systems which his diagnostic psi determined to be involved in the physical pathology. Urbanization has produced similar developments in other transitional contexts, such as Buddhism (which refines the psychological side of salvation in the elite urban context) or the modern Western elaboration of the ancient sciences of psychology. Urbanization more than anything else separates us from the primitive, since its way changes inalterably everything of the primordial world it encounters.

The more recent urban *curanderos* lack significant contact with nature, leaving behind naturalism as a base of their medical paradigm. Córdova himself realized how the cityscape had transformed the normal human condition of archaic times, and he deplored even the way many of these urban "shamans" extracted the vision vine.

Córdova's naturalism is unbelievable to current orthodoxy as indeed is all journey into the primal world—the "South Seas," for instance Melville's haphazard stumbling into the aboriginal Marquesas, as recounted in his book *Typee* (equally unbelieved in its time). Knowing the reality of the other profoundly fulfills something within us, but we always have the problem of remaining ourselves while experiencing the other. Anthropologists become painfully aware of this during their Ph.D. initiatory field research. Can one really understand the experience of the other as both observer and participant? Can anyone share reality with someone from another culture at the level of assumptions and fundamental structuring of perceptual reality (called myth)? We begin to feel a sense of unreality as if we always must see things through Robert Gardner's movie camera which in the early 1960's voraciously consumed scenes of ritual war among New Guinea highlanders.

Córdova's immersion in the aboriginal is as authentic as any on record, and gives us at least a sense of the archaic for one New World Amazonian group. Why? Because he was taken over completely, entirely re-educated to become a person of special initiatory knowledge. We see in this book how such knowledge was directed and utilized, how it worked as a scientific knowledge fully as adequate to their needs as our own is (which considers itself as exclusive possessor of valid understanding of reality, such as in medical diagnosis and treatment). How did they come to such knowledge, millennia ago, when we have just in the last centuries released our sciences from their aboriginal dark ages? We must now re-examine our knowledge and medical paradigms and temper our mechanistic medicine's cult of efficiency with the kind of naturalism don Manuel speaks of here.

This book allows us to reassess our interpretation of civilized as opposed to primitive. In *Typee*, Meville's hero Toomoo shows how difficult it has been for civilized man to approach the aboriginal other. Enmeshed in his culture's presentation of that other as primitive, cannibalistic and savage, Melville struggled mightily to rise above cultural identification, and succeeded much more than his readers, who disbelieved his account or demanded expurgations of his original *Typee* text. Not only did his era urge him to doubt his own amazed observations of savage natives, but had it not been for the appearance of his compatriot, Toby, to corroborate his story, his contemporaries may never have believed him. Córdova went far beyond this to become a master of another world's knowledge and healing ways. Only because of deep familial ties did his heart turn him away from that alien world where enemies began to threaten his life. Córdova made a journey many have dreamed of—into the mysteries from which we are separated by dense urban jungles. Córdova's life reminds me both of Gilgamesh and the image of the Buddha under the bodhi tree because all three derive from the fundamental human search for ecstatic knowledge. Gilgamesh's loss of the herb of immortality eloquently reflects the alienation of urban people from naturalism, while Buddha's vision opened an access to spirit in metaphysics and meditative practice better suited to alienated urbanites.

We usually oppose our cultural honorific, "civilized," to the primitive, considering civilization superior to the lower condition of primitive savagery or barbarism. Civilization refers to a form of socio-cultural adaptation and group survival which arose when plant and animal domesticates produced surplus power with consequent expansion of urban populations and specialization. All humans live in cultures which are strictly comparable; some recent cultures have become civilizations, but this gives no intrinsic superiority to others. Cultures which are civilized develop urban ways of life; their environment is almost entirely the production of artificial human technology. As such by their culture, civilizations then separate themselves from nature, an alienation of their own creation. So to live in civilization implies no superiority, and the status of cultural systems like medicine is independent of whether the culture is civilized or not. Civilizations may have a retarding effect, in the total picture of evolution, since their vast use of externalized power has weakened the powers of mind in civilizations—witness the loss of psi and the comparative rarity of controlled access to ecstasy. No longer does our living in civilization allow us to consider ourselves superior to our precursor human traditions. We now learn that these curious beasts from pre-Columbian times could and did behave as intelligently as we do, right down to preventive public health measures and specific treatment and control of human diseases. If we are so afraid of cannibals we must somehow be cannibalizing something ourselves, as indeed it often was, and is today, when civilization's power meets the primitive.

Córdova's life reveals something of the native we have before missed, namely its truthfulness to our sense of humanness. However, one must adopt a trans-cultural perspective to understand archaic experiences since they will not likely be easily included in the current scientific paradigm of reality. Córdova's culture relied on intuitional ecstatic knowledge and tried to harmonize with nature rather than to dominate and shape it. Somehow this threatens us. The psi access to knowledge of the physical world is excluded from our experience, for we have few initiations which would make such knowledge common rather than miraculous or magical. *Ayahuasca* is not the key, but rather the transformation which occurs in any culture when human awareness by whatever means enters into ecstatic knowing. In ancient India who bothered to remember what plant Soma really was when the way of knowledge it initiated and the psychic energy it released, samadhi, was available everywhere?

The Amazonian medicine Córdova learned was fully civil because it arose from and responded realistically to human need. It is savage (whether in civilization or not) when any person fails to seek valid knowledge and to respond to human need; supposedly we now possess the former and have left the latter trait in the lower animal realm. Responding with love and caring partakes in the essentially human. Medical care for the distressed, sick, lame and dying defines civil humanity, not whether we live in primeval forest or urban jungle. The image of Manuel Córdova's life allows us to glimpse into an ancestral age, restoring to us touch with originary humanness obscured since the planet has come to be dominated by Columbian ways. This Amazon we assume never to have risen above ignorant savagery is able to know and respond as we, with as empirical a knowledge to survive the threats of disease and annihilation in balance with nature.

Since this book concerns the meaning of the pre-Columbian world, Alfred Crosby's conclusion to his book, *The Columbian Exchange*, will well serve to introduce us to the ultimate import of the pages to follow.

> Not for half a billion years, at least, and probably for long before that, has an extreme or permanent physical change affected the whole earth. The single exception to this generality may be European man and his technologies, agricultural and industrial. He has spread all over the globe, and non-European peoples have adopted his techniques in all but the smallest islets. His effect is comparable to an increase in the influx of cosmic rays or the raising of whole new chains of Andes and Himalayas.
>
> The Columbian exchange has included man, and he has changed the Old and New Worlds sometimes inadvertently, sometimes intentionally, often brutally. It is possible that he and the plants and animals he brings with him have caused the extinction of more species of life forms in the last four hundred years than the usual processes of evolution might kill off in a million. Man kills faster than the pace of evolution: There has been no million years since Columbus for evolution to devise a replacement for the passenger pigeon. No one can remember what the pre-Columbian flora of the Antilles was like, and the trumpeter swan and the buffalo and a hundred other species have been reduced to such small numbers that a mere twitch of a change in ecology or man's wishes can eliminate them. The flora and fauna of the Old and especially of the New World have been reduced and specialized by man. Specialization almost always narrows the possibilities for future changes: for the sake of present convenience, we loot the future.
>
> The Columbian exchange has left us with not a richer but a

more impoverished genetic pool. We, all of the life on this planet, are the less for Columbus, and the impoverishment will increase.[16]

Willard Johnson
University of California at San Diego

NOTES

1. F. Bruce Lamb, *Wizard of the Upper Amazon, The Story of Manuel Córdova-Rios* (Boston: Houghton-Mifflin Company, 1974, Second Edition), p. 199.
2. In my work I use many words for the pre-Columbian world which Córdova entered in the upper Amazon, including originary, archaic, primitive, primeval, primordial, prehistoric, primal, native, aboriginal, autochthonous and indigenous, using these terms descriptively with no negative connotation. Two great temporal divides separate us from the primitive human state. First came the development of plant and animal domesticates leading to urban cultures called civilizations supported by surplus agricultural and industrial production. When agricultural societies changed the mode of human adaptation from hunting and gathering, or horticulture, or nomadic pastoralism, these forms of the first or originary mode of human livelihood came gradually to be replaced by agricultural civilizations with their urban artificial environments. The second temporal watershed came when Columbus linked the Old and the New Worlds to obscure the genuine otherness of the pre-Columbian with a European veneer, or to eradicate it altogether. As urban Columbian people we live twice removed from the world Córdova entered at the beginning of this century. For one, the Indian culture was prehistoric, archaic, rather than historical, and secondly, it was undeniably pre-Columbian.
3. F. Bruce Lamb, *Wizard of the Upper Amazon*, New York: Atheneum, 1971; as *The Stolen Chief*, London: Hale, 1972; as *Der weise Indio vom Amazonas*, Munchen: Scherz Verlag, 1982.
4. Though nearly our contemporaries in the Twentieth Century,

the Indians who trained Córdova were still living in a prior human age; thus what we learn of their epistemology and traditions can give us some sense of the pre-historic, pre-Columbian world.

5. Shamanism is the form of pre-historic culture which used controlled access to ecstatic states. Ecstasy is a non-personal knowing state, usually of ritually determined duration and context, used to acquire knowledge in ways not limited by the reach of the physical senses. Psi is a short form of psychic, indicating knowledge gained not through physical means, but through the non-physical reach of awareness. Shamans acquire psi powers through their ecstatic experience; an ecstaticant is an agent, an active placebo which changes attention and consequent mental experience. In Córdova's medicine, psi powers are not interpreted spiritually, but rather are directed to the empirical world, the jungle or the body.
6. *Economic Botany* 26 (April 1972), p. 197.
7. Others initiated into archaic knowledge have published accounts of their lives, and are relevant to our thoughts here; for example, Richard Erdoes recorded Lame Deer's remembrances in *Lame Deer Seeker of Visions, The Life of a Sioux Medicine Man* (New York: Simon and Schuster, 1972).
8. Bruce Holbrook came to similar conclusions when comparing the traditional Chinese knowledge paradigm to that of our current science (*The Stone Monkey*, New York: William Morrow, 1981), with specific reference to medical consequences.
9. Marlene Dobkin de Rios, *Visionary Vine, Psychedelic Healing in the Peruvian Amazon* (San Franciso: Chandler Publishing Company, 1972 and Prospect Heights, Illinois: Waverly, 1984).
10. For references, see her *Hallucinogens: Cross-Cultural Perspectives* (Albuquerque: University of New Mexico Press, 1984), pp. 225-226, and note her summary in Chapter 12, "Urban Amazonian Mestizos of Peru," pp. 173-189 on *ayahuasqueros*.
11. In *Medical Anthropology* 8:1 (Winter 1984), pp. 60-70.
12. Luis Eduardo Luna, "The Healing Practices of a Peruvian Shaman" and "The Concept of Plants as Teachers Among Four Mestizo Shamans of Iquitos, Northeastern Peru," *Journal of*

Ethnopharmacology 11 (1984), pp. 123-133 and 135-156.

13. *American Anthropologist* 73 (1971), pp. 742-756.
14. This draws from a widespread aboriginal Amazonian *ayahuasca* complex, as identified for instance in J. M. Cooper's 1949 contribution to the *Handbook of South American Indians* (Vol. 5) in the junction of the upper Orinoco and Amazon rivers; Plutarco Naranjo's "Hallucinogenic Plant Use and Related Indigenous Belief Systems in the Ecudorian Amazon" (*Journal of Ethnopharmacology*, 1 (1979) pp. 121-145) describes one of many individual instances of this. De Rios, *Hallucinogens* pp. 175-176, summarizes attested traditional uses of *ayahuasca*.
15. For example, compare de Rios' summary of *ayahuasca* use in her Mestizo urban Peruvian sample: "The psychoactive ayahuasca drink is used mainly to diagnose the magical causality of illness, as well as to deflect and neutralize the evil magic that is deemed responsible for certain types of illness. In no way does the drug serve as a panacea for sickness; rather it is part of a complex ritual healing ceremony." (*Hallucinogens*, p. 179).
16. Alfred W. Crosby, *The Columbian Exchange, Biological and Cultural Consequences of 1492* (Westport, Connecticut: Greenwood Press, 1972), pp. 218-219.

Foreword

The Huni Kui tribesmen in the Peruvian-Brazilian border area between the Rios Juruá and Purus long ago achieved what Drs. Timothy Leary and Richard Alpert were first seeking at Harvard during the 1960's in their experimental use of hallucinogenic substances for altering or stimulating certain functions of the mind. The Huni Kui seem to have been able, judging from Manuel Córdova's experience, to tap biological memories going back countless generations and at least to some extent to anticipate the future. Apparently, they also had developed, and used on Córdova, a practical method for the accelerated transfer of accumulated knowledge from one person to another.

These so-called primitive people, perhaps only a select group of them, found a process for focusing individual and group awareness at a deeper than conscious level, on a sphere of perception beyond the personal dimension. By the use of non-addictive psychoactive plant extracts they made contact with a transpersonal field of mental activity. The fact that this capability was restricted in its application to a limited social and cultural milieu of the Amazon forest does not at all circumscribe its potential for constructive use in other circumstances.

The shimmering golden aura evoked in the mind during a state of trance has been experienced and described by many modern observers other than Manuel Córdova. But few if any of them seem to have used the trance experience in as structured and positive a manner as Córdova, perhaps lacking his vigorous preparatory training. During this change in phase of consciousness brought on by taking the non-addictive, natural plant extracts *ayahuasca-yagé* or *chicuro piripiri* there comes a release—an intense cerebral clarity, a sense of unbounded awareness of knowledge and capacity for creativity, a feeling of peace and euphoria. When this happens the inner eye of the mind seems to open for an exploration of the interior little-used spaces of the cerebral labyrinth. There, entangled among the most elemental roots of the primordial identity in the brain stem, memories from perhaps a million years of evolution seem to await exposure and review. Sensory impressions of such subtlety that they normally go unrecorded begin to register as signals from outside the body fade and cease to dominate the brain. Latent sensory and perceptive capacities suppressed by the conscious mind thus become available, giving access to the vast collective unconscious with its untranslated body memories of both near and distant past. Perhaps on some unknown unconscious level the genetic encoder DNA provides a bridge to biological memories of all living things, an aura of unbounded awareness manifesting itself in the activated mind.

This does not mean that instant, universal erudition is available to the first acid-head who goes on a fast trip. From the information available it appears that Leary and Alpert,[1] lacking the experience and support of traditional ritual practices to control and orient the path of their experiments, failed to establish any acceptable practices and goals for their work, which ended in chaos and exile. Government agency experimentation on human beings with the hallucinogenic compounds LSD, BZ, and others—recounted on television and well documented in print—remind me that savagery and barbarism still exist in our inter-human relationships. Both Army and C.I.A. programs for testing LSD using uninformed and ill-prepared subjects have resulted in a number of deaths from sucicide. Instead of re-examining their programs in order to correct faulty practices, these organizations went to great lengths to cover up their tracks as they pressed on with their brutal, unfortunate experimentation on humans.

The use of LSD or "acid" blossomed and waned in the drug sub-culture in the 1960's, as clandestine use was stimulated by publicity on the fiasco at Harvard. There is no way to know how many deaths and ruined lives are attributable to unguided, unsupervised experimentation with this substance. One day Manuel Córdova commented on one of the newspaper accounts, saying "It seems this LSD that people in your country are using has effects very similar to those of the jungle extract of the vision vine." I told him of one young man who had described to me some of his experiences with LSD and then said he stopped using it because of the increasingly morbid and frightening reactions he got from the drug. Córdova replied without hesitation. "Of course! Without proper controls that is a typical reaction, and continued use under such conditions can ruin the mind. But with preparation, guidance, and training, the vision process can be channelled to constructive use."[2]

We have only a most primitive understanding of how the stimulated mind functions. We now seem to be dismissing the study of psychoactive substances as a source of understanding, knowledge, and enlightenment, or relegating it in America to the fragmented floundering of misguided people. There are plenty of examples from the past history of the human race to guide our efforts in seeking an understanding of how the mind functions. The ancient *soma* cults of India, perhaps for good reasons, gave up use of the hallucinogenic extract from the poisonous mushroom *Amanita muscaria* for less dangerous methods of producing similar results by fasting, contemplation, and meditation. Most of the great religious leaders of the world have also used fasting and meditation to induce meaningful insights. The superficial reacton to taking LSD, peyote, or *ayahuasca* on a casual, even a so-called experimental, basis is perhaps well enough known. However, one cannot keep from speculating on what enlightenment might develop were there to be available, within the cultural milieu of our own modern twentieth-century world, the type of indoctrination which Manuel Córdova received in an isolated Amazon jungle setting. In the Western Hemisphere there is a long tradition among indigenous peoples of using hallucinogens from many plant sources as a means of developing adjustments to harsh environments, often under a life of oppression restricted to stringent necessities. The *Handbook of South American Indians* published by the Smithsonian Institution comments only briefly on the training of a shaman among the Indians who held Córdova captive. The *Handbook* tells of the neophyte shaman learning the sorcerer's art (among Panoan tribes) by undergoing months of intense instruction, during which time he is kept insensate or in long trance states by an extract prepared from jungle plants called *honi* (*ayahuasca* in Quechua). In contrast, the detailed descriptions given by Manuel

Córdova of the meticulous preparation and indoctrination to which he was subjected are a priceless revelation.

Perhaps Córdova's experiences with *ayahuasca,* when as a very young man he was plunged into the frightening and strange new world of the Huni Kui tribesmen, may exemplify and point the way to legitimate use of psychotropic or psychedelic substances. After that long indoctrination and years of practice in the use of mind-stimulating plant extracts, Córdova was able to achieve his diagnostic and healing goals without the use of these substances that seem to have activated otherwise unused capacities of his mind. The channels, open and well established, were then available when he needed them.

These events in Córdova's life came to my attention while we collaborated on a timber survey in the tropical forests of the Peruvian Amazon. Late one afternoon early in our project we pulled our motor launch up to a small clearing in the riverbank jungle. Here a group of palm-thatched huts marked a place on the Rio Tigre called Pavayacu. During the short tropical dusk after our evening meal Don Manuel and I sat talking on deck; in the forest nearby a *panguana* or tinamous (small jungle partridge) sounded its mournful four-note call for a sleeping mate. An answer came from far off in another direction, and the calls echoed back and forth in the gathering darkness. The conversation between us stopped and a faraway look came over Córdova's expressive face.

"You hear that *panguana* calling? It reminds me of a time in my youth over fifty years ago when I awaited nightfall alone in a forest *caucho* camp."

From that point on, during the fifteen years I knew Manuel Córdova, he continued to stretch my understanding of the place of man in nature as he told me about his life in the Amazon forest where he searched for knowledge of its wonders and for ways of utilizing its boundless resources.

The first chapter in what follows is included here primarily for those who have not read my book *Wizard of the Upper Amazon* which contains a detailed account of how Manuel Córdova acquired his extensive knowledge of herbal medicine and learned the secrets of healing. This chapter will also serve as a foreshadowing of Córdova's path through untapped states of consciousness to unique kinds of esoteric knowledge that have a role in relieving human suffering.

F. B. L.
Santa Fe, New Mexico

1

Ayahuasca

Between daylight and dark in the tropical forest the brief dusk brings on an interesting change of scene. There on the deck of our motor launch at Pavayacu on the Rio Tigre, the call of a bird prompted Manuel Córdova to speak. He began with an account of his days as a rubber cutter in the Amazon forest.

THE HAUNTING MELANCHOLY CALL OF A *YUNGURURU*, A LARGE JUNGLE partridge, floated on the still evening air from the forest nearby and off in the depths of the jungle came a faint reply that I could barely distinguish. A lingering sense of foreboding clouded my thoughts as I built up our cooking fire to help dispel the gathering gloom of night. I had been left for the day to guard our jungle *caucho*[1] camp on the upper Rio Juruá.

So far as I know my companions never returned. That night I spent miserably alone in camp. Early the next morning I went to a nearby creek to draw a bucket of water. Glancing up from the stream at an unexpected sound, I found myself surrounded by Indians with strange designs painted on their naked bodies. Each stood poised with an arrow or lance drawn and ready for the slightest show of resistance from me. So we stood for a long frozen moment held by the magnetism of our staring eyes.

Before the spell broke one of them came to my side, took the bucket and removed a knife from my belt. At a hand signal my rifle was removed from where I had leaned it against a tree. Then two of them came and tied my hands behind my back. During all this their communication consisted only of hand and facial signals. I could have resisted, fought with them. But to what avail at odds of fifteen to one, and with the advantage of surprise on their side?

On a command which I could not understand, we all returned to the camp. There, while two stood guard beside me, the others took the camp apart. It was all directed by one man and was well organized. Everything useful was quickly arranged into pack loads. The half-roasted partridge I had put over the fire was portioned out and gulped down quickly. I was given some and I forced myself to eat it, against an unknown future. Our camp shelters went up in flames.

During all this my mind was a hurricane of thoughts, trying to understand what was happening while at the same time searching for something I could do. At one moment I thought surely my companions would return and let go with a fusillade of rifle shots at these savages and set me free. But then I realized all of our firearms were accounted for in the equipment being collected into pack loads. Where were my friends? Had the Indians kept them from coming in last night? What had been done to them? And what were the plans for my future? We had heard stories of cannibals in this area. What chance of escape might there be?

I looked around at the Indians and noticed that my guards were intently watching every move I made, even a turning of my head. All of these men, though not large, seemed well built, muscular. Their movements were smooth and purposeful. Each one was naked except for a belt or band at the waist.

Now my captors formed a single line with me in the middle, the men immediately in front and behind me obviously responsible for my actions. Then we were off through the forest, leaving the camp a smoldering ruin.

As we left and during the first few hours I kept track of the direction of travel. The sun was over my left shoulder, so it was southwest we were going. There was no sign of a trail that I could see, but the pace was fast. The Indians seemed to glide through the forest without effort, while vines and thorns were constantly pulling at me. It was especially difficult for me with my hands tied. I needed them for balance. But from the first moment my instinct had been to show no sign of weakness or emotion, and I kept up somehow.

We maintained a southwesterly direction up and down hills through rolling country. I tried to keep track of the small streams we crossed, as landmarks, but with the exertion of our pace I soon lost track. In the forest the sunlight seldom reached the ground, so it was cool, but with the high humidity and the exertion of trying to keep up I was constantly in a running sweat.

As the pace of travel kept on without let-up I became less and less aware of the details of my surroundings. By mid-afternoon I was exhausted and, even with extreme effort, was stumbling as I walked.

We stopped by a small stream and my hands were untied. By example they indicated that I should wash and rinse my mouth. But when I gulped the water instead of rinsing my mouth, they led me away from the stream. I was dying of thirst, but they would let me have no more water. Pieces of smoked meat were passed around. Mine was so dry I could hardly swallow it, but I knew I had to eat to survive and forced it down.

After only a short time my hands were tied again and we were off. The food helped, and strength to go on came from some reserve, perhaps in the mind. This time it was for all night. As dusk deepened into darkness the pace slowed somewhat to accomodate my difficulties, but we did not stop until daylight.

Stopping again at a small stream, I followed gestured instructions, rinsing my mouth out and swallowing only a small amount of water in spite of my desire to gulp it down. They allowed me to bathe. My body was covered with scratches from a thousand thorns along the way and my clothes were in tatters. The pause was only a brief one, and we were soon walking again at the forced pace of the day before. This we kept up for another day and another night!

I was near the point of collapse from exhaustion after these two days and two nights of almost continuous forced march. For the last few hours before dawn on the third day I was barely staggering forward. As it was getting light we came up a small hill and stopped. Here my captors opened a well-hidden deposit of supplies. I collapsed on the ground in an agony of fatigue. Even breathing seemed an effort beyond my power. I was in fact barely conscious, my mind able to develop only the most fragmented bits of thought: Where? . . . How? . . . Why? . . .

After several hours of tortured rest and fitful sleep I was prodded into eating and was given a small clay dish of thick sour liquid to drink. This proved to be refreshing and stimulating, and I felt as if I were coming painfully back to life.

Late in the afternoon two Indians came into camp from the direction of our arrival and seemed to report, with many gestures, to the leader. This must have been a rear guard who had been checking to see if we had been followed. I knew that we had not been, for even if one or more of my companions had escaped and gone for help, it would take days to reach the nearest settlement. And the possibility of their survival seemed very unlikely. The Indians also must have been satisfied, because we rested on through the night, but they did not build a fire.

Before dark one of my guards rubbed crushed leaves of a small shrub on my scratches and cuts, which relieved the itching and pain and also stopped the bleeding. This was done without any show of favor or feeling.

As soon as the sun went down, moisture from the high humidity in the air began to condense on the leaves and was soon dripping from the treetops with a constant patter that continued all night. For protection against this cold dripping dew, the Indians put up individual palm-leaf shelters on stick frames. They were only large enough to sit in, and mine was surrounded by others—with no avenue of escape. It was a night of cold, misery, pain and fear that I will never forget. My whole body ached from unbelievable exertion and I was emotionally shattered by events. My thoughts were still fragmentary and disconnected—mostly of the past. But what of the future? A formless void to be filled by events still undreamed of. I had heard plenty of Indian stories in the villages and camps we had visited on the way to the Juruá. Storytelling was a pastime. But reality in all that I had heard was unclear.

I was prodded from a troubled sleep at dawn. All evidence of our camp was carefully scattered before we set out again. We stopped at the first stream for a bath, and then the march was on again—still southwest, but at a more moderate pace now. The Indians seemed released from the first pressure of escape from the area of their attack.

I tried to keep track of the days, and I tried to observe the country. I knew that the Rio Juruá was to our right, for we had crossed no major river. It was up and down hills, over fallen trees, through swamps and small streams. Compared to the grueling pace of the first two days and nights, this part of the journey was mild. We stopped every night to rest and traveled only from dawn to dusk.

One day it was cloudy and rainy all day. The forest was eerie, shrouded in whitish mist. The rain was filtered through the foliage starting 150 feet above our heads. The air was heavy, completely saturated with moisture. Every leaf and twig discharged its load of accumulated moisture if touched. This was the kind of day when caucheros stayed in camp, mended their clothes, ate and talked.

On what by my count was the ninth day of travel, I noticed about noon one of the Indians rejoining the line with a small forest deer slung over his shoulder. Later another appeared with two game birds. This was the first hunting I had noticed on the trip. The feeling among the Indians this morning had been different somehow—faces less severe and some conversation back and forth. The pace had definitely picked up again.

About mid-afternoon I saw off to the left a momentary break in the forest, a whole big patch of blue sky. Soon after we passed by what was obviously a cultivated patch of *yuca.*

We must be nearing a village, I thought. What would the end of the journey bring? Why had these Indians not already killed me? I was quite sure they had killed one, if not all, of my cauchero companions.

The way now led up a long hill. Suddenly there was a loud squawking of macaws and almost immediately we stepped into a village clearing filled with naked Indians—men, women and children. They crowded around and pushed one another for a better view. There was an immediate hubbub of chattering that stopped abruptly when a thin, ancient, long-haired old man stepped calmly through the throng. He came up to where I stood, my hands still tied behind my back, and deliberately looked me over.

I looked back at him just as deliberately. I saw a very old man with a distinct Oriental cast to his face. A feathered headband held back a shock of reddish-brown hair that came to the middle of his back. A few long yellowish whiskers on his upper lip and chin added to the Oriental look. And whereas every other Indian in sight was naked, he wore a simple sleeveless garment of coarse white cotton that came almost to his bony knees. This, I knew, must be the chief.

From the moment of my arrival there this ancient and wizened headman took complete charge of every detail of my existence in this strange place. After the confusion from the first hullabaloo of my arrival, there seemed to be no menace in the attitude of these Indians toward me. Within a day or two the old chief started efforts to communicate with me. These were halting at first since I understood not a word of their language.

As I recovered from being transplanted to this primitive society and became adjusted to the simple life style in the nude, new elements in the part I was expected to play began to emerge. It soon became evident that they did not expect to eat me as I at first supposed. The old chief put me on a restricted diet, purged my body with herbal concoctions which I was given to drink, and then bathed me in medicinal preparations that caused at first a feverish reaction, then one of nervous tension, and later a feeling of calm well-being.

One afternoon a group of men gathered around the chief and me. They had strange designs painted in red on their faces. With instructions from the chief they proceeded to paint my face also. When this was done to their satisfaction a soft chant started, led by the chief, and we marched calmly off into the forest on a dim trail. Soon we came to a small clearing in the forest undergrowth by a trickling stream. One of the men lighted a fire. Four others withdrew to the edge of our opening in the jungle and took up guard positions. The chief sounded a birdcall and an answer came back from several directions off in the forest.

With a change in the tone and rhythm of the chant the old man put a bundle of leaves on the fire and a billowing cloud of fragrant smoke rose into the vaulted structure created by the branches of the giant trees around us. Holding a fan of brilliant feathers the chief enveloped us all in the cloud of smoke which produced a spell of tranquility among the group. Momentarily all sounds of the forest seemed suspended. A warm glow of late afternoon sunlight filtered through a small gap in the vegetation and then faded.

The mood changed with a new chant as the chief dipped into an earthenware pot and filled a small gourd cup for each of us. The men all held cups as if to drink and I did likewise with a fleeting momentary thought that I should resist. We drank in unison. I sensed a bitter taste to the greenish concoction but had no other immediate reaction. Then we all calmly sat down at a motioned direction from our leader and waited as the chanting continued. The animation of the song picked up and soon I felt a violent seizure go through my body. From that moment on I had very little recollection of my first session with *ayahuasca*.[2]

The next morning with shafts of sunlight filtering through the forest canopy I woke from a troubled sleep. The group gathered around, encouraging my return to consciousness. After swallowing a gourd full of mush made from ground-up fruit I felt better. Soon we started on our way back to the village. There, as the people gathered around, everyone seemed solicitous of my condition. At this time I noticed a subtle change in my perception. Even though I could still not speak their language I understood a great deal more of what they said to me or between themselves in my presence.

This session with *ayahuasca* was only the beginning. The old chief, whose name was Xumu (Dominator), started again putting me through a regimen of strict diet and purges. When this was completed to his satisfaction, Xumu took me alone one day to a small clearing in the forest near the village. Here he said to me, "You drink alone this time, but I will be here to guide you. Every reaction to your preparation has been favorable. Drink now from this cup and be ready for profound and pleasing visions that will come to you. There is much in the forest that you do not sense or understand. This will change. You must know *all* to be the channel and lead our hunters in the visions to improve their search for food in the forest."

He gave me a cup of liquid to drink the same as before. Then, in our hammocks swung close together between the trees, we lay back and I awaited the reaction I had learned to expect . . . a pleasant feeling of euphoria . . . a soft pulsating hum in my ear. This sound seemed to float off up into the tree tops. My eyes followed the sound. As my glance wandered among the branches of the forest canopy I became intricately aware of the unimaginable beauty in the details of texture in the leaves and branches. A birdsong floated down from the tree tops, exquisite and shimmering, almost visible in its intensity. Each note of the cascading song I could suspend and savor as I desired. A movement of cool air rustled the leaves and created an ecstasy of sensation as it bathed my skin.

The old chief sensed my mental state and spoke in a low tone: "Visions come." At the sound of his sonorous voice all barriers between us melted away. We were as one, united it seemed through some telepathic code of ancient man or universal knowing. Then with evocative, descriptive chants and in other ways I cannot explain, Chief Xumu brought visions into my mind of all the birds and animals of the forest. Events in the daily lives and habitats of each appeared to me in infinite detail at his suggestion.

Late in the afternoon he gave me another gourd cupful of the vision extract to drink, saying "We have night work to do." With the almost instant effect of this draught so soon after the first, a passing firefly lit up the deep shadows of the forest with a brilliance seeming to approach the light of day. My sensitivity of hearing picked up sounds of which I had been formerly unaware. In this state of heightened perception the slightest stimulus produced reactions of overwhelming intensity. "You will learn to see and hear at night like an owl," the chief said to me—and already it was so. With chants and calls of various animals Xumu evoked in my visions vivid episodes in the lives of the nocturnal inhabitants of our forest. All became a part of my knowledge. On awakening in the morning from a strange sleep it seemed I was returning from a distant journey to unknown, unremembered places. And still this was only the beginning.

The old man led me through a long series of similar training sessions with only a short day or two of rest between. On these days Xumu took me to the forest to reinforce my experience in the visions. With all this I became nervous and afraid of going insane. The chief noticed and took pains to reassure me that as long as I followed his diets and other instructions I had nothing to fear. As this training under the spell of *ayahuasca* progressed I noticed an acceleration in my thought processes and a developing sense of clairvoyance. By focusing my attention on an individual I could anticipate his actions, plans, and purposes. Xumu observed this and was pleased, telling me that my power to foresee events and know the future would improve. He told me all this was necessary to protect and control the tribe. It became evident that the role of leadership eventually would pass to me.

When some hunter had a stretch of bad luck and could not feed his family he would come to tell his troubles to the chief. Then a call would go out to the best hunters and detailed instructions given to prepare for a vision session. In a few days after the conditions set down by the chief had been fulfilled we would go to our secluded spot in the forest. By taking together the magic extract of the vine they called *honi*[3] (that we call *ayahuasca*), and led by Xumu's chants and songs, we shared extraordinary visions of each forest animal's life, exposed to us from the combined experience of each hunter and perhaps that of their ancestors. Among us there developed an intense feeling of group awareness at some deep level of understanding. Afterward, one could only wonder about the source and profound effect of our joint reactions; even the unsuccessful hunter found that his hunting prowess had improved.

Under the guidance of Chief Xumu and using his traditional chants with their associated trains of thought, I began to attain control of the vision process. At this time we began an examination of the forest plants and their medicinal values. In great detail he showed me each plant and how to use it, alone and in combination with others. Actually, using the vision process, I felt that I was receiving the accumulated wisdom of many generations of ancestral forest dwellers, tapping biological wisdom from some source unknown.

Inevitably this old man, who had planned my capture and then meticulously engineered and controlled my training, died, thus leaving a void in the tribal life which I had to fill. But my ancestral ties did not have their origin among such primitives—at least not of the Western Hemisphere. The family relationships of my youth back in Iquitos before my capture by the Donowan clan of the Huni Kui[4] had been strong. Therefore when, several years after the death of the old chief, visions of tragedy at home in Iquitos intruded with overwhelming urgency into the clairvoyant channels of my mind, I felt impelled to take advantage of the first chance which came to escape.

The opportunity came only after spending over seven years with the Huni Kui. On a trip to trade *caucho* we had produced, I arrived at a rubber trading outpost on the Rio Purus on the border between Peru and Brazil just at the time when a supply launch prepared to depart down river to Manaus. On sudden impluse I boarded the launch to Manaus and from there went up the Amazon to my home in Iquitos. On arrival I discovered that most of my family (as seen in my visions) had recently died from an epidemic of what was called then the Spanish influenza.

Soon I found out that what I had learned living with the Indians in the forest had application outside that ancient society. A good example is my subsequent work with the Lamisto Indians producing *curare* extract for sale to the pharmaceutical trade in New York. My *ayahuasca* vision sessions with a group of Lamisto[5] from Chazúta set the stage for successful production of exportable *curare* extract—a feat many others had failed to accomplish.

2

Men of Chazúta

You have seen that wild country on the Amazon side of the cordillera on your flights over the Andes from Lima to Iquitos. The Amazon River rises in those jungle-covered sharp ridges and deep canyons almost always shrouded in mist. *Cejas de la montaña* (eyebrows of the mountains) they call that country, and well named too. Sometimes in clear weather you can see down into those dark shadowy canyons, but more often drifting clouds obscure the view. From the air only an occasional fleeting glimpse is possible into the wild inaccessible country where the men of Chazúta dwell.

Going into that country from the mountain town of Tarapoto I received a warning about the local Indians. I had already decided that the small jungle village of Chazúta fit into my *curare* production plans. When my friends in Tarapoto found this out they warned me: "*Tenga cuidado, los hombres de Chazúta son temibles hechiceros todos* (Be careful, the men of Chazúta are feared sorcerers every one)." Sorcerers, if you know how to deal with them, can be useful. Also, I knew before going there that the forests of the country around Chazúta had a greater abundance of the jungle vine *ampihuasca*[1] (poison vine) than any other known part of the Amazon region. Forest-dwelling Indians make from this vine a lethal arrow and blowgun dart poison called by some "winged death," better known as *curare*.

Word reached us that the substance had value outside the Amazon. In delicate surgical operations the purified extract can be used to relax selected strategic muscles of a patient during critical moments of a surgeon's work. My employers had commitments to certain New York pharmaceutical firms to provide the raw jungle extract for laboratory purification, which would then be made available to surgeons when needed. But efforts to produce a suitable jungle extract on a commercial scale had failed.

The person who first attempted to produce this *curare* was a friend of mine, and we often discussed his efforts before sudden death terminated his work. From his comments I was convinced that he had not been careful enough during the extraction process in his jungle camp. Now the turn of fortune involved me in this same dangerous enterprise. But I had my own protection from my training at the hand of old Izidoro, one of the best Ticuna Indian *curare* makers in the whole upper Amazon. That experience of years ago still remained vivid in my mind.

The men of Chazúta of whom I hoped to make allies belonged to the Lamisto tribe. To escape Inca tyranny and the brutal Spanish *conquistadores* these Indians several hundred years ago moved down from the high Andes plateau into the forbidding lands of the *cejas de la montaña.* Superstitious and clannish people, they do not welcome outsiders. Yet in their territory the *ampihuasca* vine grows best. And if I was not to fail in the production of a commercial *curare* extract I needed the help of the Lamisto.

In spite of the warning about the feared sorcerers who lived there, Chazúta seemed to me to provide the best site to establish my influence among these potentially unfriendly people. The strategic location and special reputation of the Chazutinos to the rest of the Lamisto in the region as sorcerers gave Chazúta significance to my plans. In the almost impassable jumble of steep mountain ridges and narrow canyons the Lamisto villages are small and scattered far apart. You get to them on foot or by mule back. There is no other way to reach these isolated places.

On my first trip to Chazúta from Tarapoto, which has an airport, Chuquizuta guided my way. He had come to Tarapoto on a trading mission, and since I spoke to him in his own dialect he agreed to take me to Chazúta. Along the trail on our way I noticed throughout the forest the vine *ayahuasca*—vine of the spirits. It was well-known to me for the vision extract it contained. But when I asked Chuquizuta if he knew the famous plant he looked at me in a strange way before answering. That gave me an idea for getting close to the Chazutinos.

"*Hie pani Taita* (Great Holy Father)," they exclaimed when I arrived and they found out that I spoke their Quechua dialect from the Andes. By talking with them in their own idiom I managed to head off much of the antipathy they might otherwise have felt toward me and my project of producing *curare* extract. I soon found out that they also knew about the spirit vine—*ayahuasca*. But from our discussions I could tell that their understanding of its use was superficial. They believed that the strong purging effect of drinking the extract cleansed their bodies and attracted useful forest spirits to help them in their hunting expeditions. The disorganized visions they saw were only incidental to them. When I suggested that *ayahuasca* visions had meaning beyond their understanding, it aroused their curiosity. They agreed to take it with me to see if what I said was true. Feared as they were by some, the sorcerers of Chazúta compliantly let themselves be persuaded to drink with me the vision vine extract *ayahuasca* that I myself prepared. I knew it would put them under my control.

Late one afternoon when the weather signs were favorable for a calm rainless night, I led a small select group in single file from their village, Chazúta, through the jungle to a place I had made ready in the forest. On the way I chanted in their dialect a simple song to hold their attention and relieve any fears or tensions they might feel.

great forest
dwelling place of our forefathers
benevolent protector of our lives
watch over us
green mantle
source of our sustenance
shelter for the spirits
of our ancestors
now watch over us

When we reached the opening I had cleared in the undergrowth beneath a canopy of large forest trees beside a small stream, I kindled a small fire, continuing my chant. Deliberately and calmly I arranged my companions in a circle around the fire. Late afternoon bird songs floated down from the tree tops. A shaft of filtered sunlight momentarily illumined our gathering place with a friendly glow. As the sunlight faded and the fire became our source of light, sounds of the night, which comes suddenly in the deep forest, took over the aural background of our scene. Then I asked those Lamisto Indians of Chazúta to remove their clothing, proceeding to set the example myself. Thus we removed all that separated and restrained our bodies from the most direct contact with the ambience of this forest place. We shed our inhibitions with our shirts and pants, becoming simpler, more natural beings—better attuned to the dark and brooding forest. Our naked bodies glowed in the fire light.

Chanting again, I put a bundle of leaves on the fire.

> fragrant leaves
> tranquil smoke
> prepare our minds
> for visions to come

A billowing white cloud of pungent, fragrant smoke from the burning leaves floated up into the tree tops, enveloping us at the same time in the spell of its aroma. A trance-like tranquility prevailed as we breathed in the fragrant smoke.

My chanting held their attention as I poured out into small gourd cups a greenish-brown liquid which I had prepared several days earlier: sections of the vision vine I had boiled with the leaves of a certain shrub I found in the forest.

> magic vine of the forest
> leaves of the shrub
> with markings of the boa
> bring us visions
> bring us awareness
> give us knowledge
> of our forest home

As we drank together the potion in our cups I noticed a slightly bitter taste and wondered momentarily about the strength of this *ayahuasca*. Plants even of the same species vary from one region to another and there had been no time to test the strength of the local variety here at Chazúta. That it was certainly strong enough soon became apparent.

One of the first reactions to a strong dose of *ayahuasca* is a violent discharge of energy through the nervous system. This can be a traumatic experience for imbibers untrained to control the reaction mentally. The Chazutinos had told me they took this vision vine purge and I assumed they had some control. This conclusion on my part turned out to be erroneous, at least in connection with the extract I was accustomed to preparing and using. Perhaps they made up a milder potion for their hunting purge.

If body condition and mental control are inadequate the individual reactions vary according to the state of the nervous system of each person. Some have violent abdominal convulsions, others experience intense nausea, and still others erotic stimulation of the whole glandular system involved with sexual response. And now suddenly, a few minutes after drinking our potion came characteristically deep and powerful reactions, violent reactions, of naked Indians. Some were loudly crapping, pissing and vomiting in the small stream beside our clearing. Others stood displaying with amazement their tremendous hard-ons. Any personal inhibitions to such manifestations had been dissolved by that first surge of response to the extract.

But these outward physical reactions lasted only a few minutes and with suggestive chanting and gestures I calmly assembled and seated them around the fire again with their eyes closed. At first, as the initial stimulus subsided, a general feeling of euphoria spread through the group, indicated by the play of expression on the usually-impassive Indian faces, and I knew they were seeing in their minds, as I was, strange formless moving visions. These multicolored blobs gradually cohered in the more formal shapes of natural forms—vague arabesque traceries of a butterfly wing, then a delicate spider web set against a subtle changing background of greenish-blue color. With evocative songs, imitated jungle sounds, and subtle gestures creating an atmosphere suitable for auto-suggestion I brought into our joint visions scenes of the forest where birds of brilliant plumage and rare song were followed by game birds, then by the hunters—the hawks and owls. In my carnivorous parade the giant harpy, the monkey-eating eagle with flaming yellow eyes and scimitar beak, was followed by the hideous but brilliantly colorful king vulture and the giant condor of the Andes. A snake-eating hawk doing battle with a fer-de-lance or yellow beard then started a procession of snakes through our visions, with the appearance of the giant *shushupi*, the bushmaster. Fire flashed from the *shushupi's* tongue and eyes, and a pulsating bluish scrollwork floated upright along his spine. Loud hissing and vicious strikes at an invisible prey accompanied his passage. Last came the enormous anaconda or boa, known to the Indians as *yacumama* or mother-of-the-water, now released onto land from its native rivers and lakes. As this incredible reptile moved slowly through the forest, every segment of the intricate pattern in his scaly hide glowed in brilliant contrasting colors.

A cool breeze passing gently through the forest carried the fragrance of night-blooming orchids from the tree tops. The combination of the cooling effect on our naked bodies and the heavy aroma in our nostrils created indescribably erotic sensations. They surged into all the sensing mechanisms of our minds. The breeze increased to a strong wind and the great trees of the forest began to sway and groan. Wild cries of unknown creatures filled the turbulent air, and the agitated vegetation roared. But this storm subsided as quickly as it had arisen. In its aftermath I brought forth a complete precisely textured series of forest animals, ending finally with a family of big spotted cats. Before my companions drifted into a troubled sleep I turned their minds loose to float through subtly colored and moving spirals and arabesques of infinite variety themselves gradually fading into the ever nothingness that surrounds and impinges on our world of light and form.

With the cacophony of morning bird song and the shafting rays of sunshine penetrating our secluded jungle glade there beside the small sparkling stream, my phantom-viewing companions gradually awakened. They looked at one another with guarded glances and conversed in whispers, verifying by their half-heard remarks that they had all witnessed the same fantastic parade of visionary birds and animals. They looked in my direction with awe and deference. I stirred up the fire and encouraged them with casual remarks to return to the world of ordinary everyday life.

When my quiet and subdued new friends had all awakened I reminded them of what had happened in those first moments after they drank properly prepared *ayahuasca*. I explained that their reactions were so violent because they had failed to follow my instructions for getting ready, especially by their not avoiding contaminating foods. I told them that if they would spend a few days with me, doing exactly as I instructed in the matter of fasting and other preparations, I would show them even more marvelous things, far beyond the revelations of the visions just ended. Shaking their heads questioningly and grinning shyly at one another in disbelief they agreed to try.

When we went back to the village I kept these men together in one hut and there among us we discussed the natural world. We talked about this land in which they lived, the eyebrows of the mountain; we examined the production of *curare* and a thousand other things. I arranged for one of the women to bring us only fresh fruit, roast chicken, and boiled white *yuca* (manioc) to eat. That first reaction to my *ayahuasca* had purged them almost completely, but I did prepare a mild extract of *achuni sacha,*[2] a nerve stimulant, to tune their systems for the visions to come.

The sun was not far from setting on the third day of our fasting when we went again to our secluded spot in the forest. This time there was a feeling of eagerness and a desire for more active participation. The men had a better idea of what to expect and were keyed up to see if I could make good my promise of fantastic unison visions. Again, as we approached the little clearing, I chanted to the forest; again, the song to the fragrant leaves as I placed the green branches on the small fire; then, pouring the liquid into the cups, I intoned the chant of the vision-vine and we prepared the medicine.

We drank together. With great mental concentration and compelling song I held their attention safely through the stage of violent reaction. Some jerked with slight muscle spasm and I knew from these signs that soon I would possess them all in the visions that were to come. Again, through evocative chants and imitation of jungle sounds and even more subtle channels of suggestion, I maintained control of the flow of visions through our collective consciousness. Beginning with changing, flowing abstract color forms of great plasticity and variety I brought into our minds scenes of the forest, giant trees and other plants, and, again, the passing parade of birds and animals.

From our long, meandering conversations of the last three days I found that these men greatly admired the spotted jaguar. This was the largest animal in their forest, and I knew that some of them were clever at trapping these uncanny beasts. So, as our fantasy progressed, to impress them I brought into our visions the shuffling, giant, big-headed spotted cat of old Chief Xumu's visions from years before in a faraway jungle with a different group of even more primitive Indians. Now as we watched him in wonder, this huge cat stumbled through the trees, grunting to himself, his tongue lolling out, his great curved fangs clearly visible. He looked harmless enough in spite of his size, until with a sudden lashing switch of his tail he became instantly and viciously alert—flashing eyes and menacing growl. From my seated companions came a collective audible response, a gasp of indrawn breath, in anticipation of some disaster. But the mighty beast of our fantasy faded from the visioned forest, to be followed by another jaguar, a magnificent black one. He reared up and tested his large curved claws on a great tree trunk, scattering bark chips in all directions, switching his tail and rumbling a growl low in his throat. Coming down to four feet again he turned with twitching tail and sprayed the scratched tree with panther piss, marking his territory. As on previous occasions when this beast had come into my visions, I had the impression—and it now also became part of my companions' visions—that I was myself merged in some strange way with this black jaguar and that we traveled as one through this forest of our dreams. All the mysteries and secrets of the jaguar world were mine. My sensing faculties became those of the black animal. Sound, sight, smell, feel and instinct were tuned in with those of this most astute beast of the forest. And we prowled together—investigating dark hidden things beyond the ken of uninitiated man, unexplainable in his language.

With the black cat fading into the forest shadows came a change in mood; there developed views of distant picturesque landscapes and strange cloud formations. Out of the clouds there strode a caravan of giant human figures in white hooded robes. In slow succession they passed among us, chanting, and each one as he passed laid a hand momentarily on each of our heads. This event was accompanied by an incandescent glow of light and an almost unbearable flow of heat through our bodies. As these apparitions faded back into the clouds from whence they came, pleasant images of colored forms took over—giant double rainbows arching and moving between clouds and accompanied by celestial music. Then this too faded into nowhere as I gradually relaxed my mental control and the phantom-viewers dozed into their fitful slumber.

Soon the morning sun and the usual forest sounds brought us back to the world of reality. And again my companions displayed their feelings of awe. All of them had drunk *ayahuasca* before my arrival, if what they had told me was true, but none had participated in anything at all like the experience we had just been through together. They spoke especially of the forest cats we had seen and seemed to shudder at the thought of meeting one of them alive. And these Indians of Chazúta assured me that *jamás habían pensado que una purga tenía tanto poder para dejarles tan lelos de todo lo que ellos sabían, y quedaron muy maravillados del poder del ayahuasca bien perparado*—never had they thought that a purge could have such power to leave them as simpletons for all they knew, and now they recognized the marvelous power of *ayahuasca* properly prepared and controlled by a master of the art.

"I sense, my friend," Córdova said to me, "that you find it difficult to grasp the significance of the influence that a *maestro ayahuasquero* has over the minds of a group of people who participate with him in a vision session of the kind I have described. This power once exerted, though perhaps subtle in its effect, does not easily disappear. As you know, in my youth I was held in its spell for several years.

"In your country, from what I read in the newspapers, people are taking something called LSD which seems to have a similar effect on the mind. Unfortunately, from the accounts I have seen this new medicine is taken in a haphazard way, more for quick thrills than trained wisdom. *Ayahuasca* is taken that way here also. But such is a dangerous pastime. What I have described to you—group visions under controlled conditions, with an experienced leader to bring out simultaneous reactions—is an affair of an entirely different order with long-lasting influences on the mind. And still all this is only a token of the profound secrets to be revealed by *ayahuasca*."

3

Rio Tigre

The need for a timber survey first brought me into this still strange, primitive world of Manuel Córdova. At the time, the euphonious names, *ayahuasca*, Chazúta, *ampihuasca*, were mere exotic additions to the spare and secular vocabulary of a newcomer to the Peruvian Amazon. But they represented things only peripheral to my purpose, having no pertinent relationship to commercial timber. During my first flight over the Andes I had looked down from the plane into the "eyebrows of the mountains" as onto an unknown planet, but my main interest then had been to determine the distribution and navigability of the rivers, for they provided the only access to most of the forest area which I had to examine. I existed predominantly in the modern world, with its physical, quantitative boundaries.

From Iquitos I went first to the Rio Tigre to begin my forest survey. A local company cooperating in the project assigned Manuel Córdova to assist me in extracting from the jungle the information I required for my survey. For this coincidence I consider myself vastly fortunate. By motor launch we navigated up the Amazon from Iquitos to the Rio Marañon and then up the Rio Tigre. We had been on the river a little more than a week when we pulled up early one morning to a palm-thatched *tambito* in a small riverbank clearing at a place called Santa Elena. No one was home and the ashes of the cooking fire were cold, but the location provided convenient access to a section of forest we wanted to examine. We tied our motor launch to a dead tree in front of the *tambito* and left the cook to explain our presence if the owner returned while we were in the forest. Then Don Manuel and I took our canoe and went into the jungle by way of a small creek. Its wandering waters led us into the hinterland through a tunnel of tropical high forest that completely shaded the stream.

Several hours later when we returned, the residents of Santa Elena had come home. The owner of the *tambito* had with him a friend who had come down from one of the upper tributaries of the Rio Tigre, the Rio Pucacuro. Since we had not gone this far up country, we were interested in asking about the composition of the forest that way. We got very little information out of him except for a rambling story about a Señor Ramírez from Iquitos who a few years past had established a camp up the Pucacuro, to explore for a source of chewing gum base produced by the *leche caspi*[1] tree and for rosewood[2] trees in order to extract their fine oil.

One day, our informant told us, a group of ten or twelve small Indians came wandering into this camp out of the forest. They were only about five feet tall, completely naked, smiling and gesturing but unable to speak Spanish. Señora Ramírez in surprise and fear at this strange visitation got a shotgun and was about to shoot into the chattering group when her husband returned to camp. He put the gun away before anyone got hurt.

Ramírez found out after much effort that these Indians could speak and understand a few words of Quechua, language of the Andes. They were Taushiros, who wander around in the forest between Peru and Equador. They had no villages but lived entirely on food gathered from the forest, moving around from one temporary camp to another.

The Ramírez family made them welcome after the near-shooting episode, and gave them food and a machete or two. This made the Indians very happy. They wandered in and out of camp from a few small palm shelters built nearby in the forest. In a few days two or three were coughing and had runny noses. Soon the others were in the same condition; by that time the first who had gotten sick were dead. The rest were quickly getting worse, flushed in the face, crying, choking, with noses and throats all stopped up. Finally those who were able wandered into the forest again. Who knows if any of them lived to continue their nomadic life? "Better never to have seen the white man," our story-teller informed us emphatically. And that was all we learned about the forests of the Rio Pucacuro.

The story finished, the two Indians there on the riverbank at Santa Elena withdrew to one side, speaking a language I could not understand. They left me to ponder the barely veiled innuendo of the sad story we had just been told. The point of it seemed clear enough: interlopers to the Rio Tigre like ourselves had little to offer but destruction. Córdova, though, was no interloper. To the surprise of our reluctant hosts he entered the animated conversation, an exchange which continued for several minutes and ended abruptly. Then the two Indians went into the shelter, picked up their machetes, and stepped into a canoe at the river bank. Soon they had disappeared into the thick vegetation that overhangs the banks of all tropical rivers.

Córdova turned and explained to me that the man from the Pucacuro had come to consult with his friend about how to cure a siege of intolerable back aches that afflicted him. Now they had gone to the forest to collect *ayahuasca* and *yagé*[3] with which they were going to brew a potion for a vision session. Tonight they would drink it and consult with the spirits of *ayahuasca* to determine the best cure for the man's malady. Córdova said to me that he had some experience in such affairs, as his stories had already revealed. Now he would like to stay and participate.

Intrigued by the prospect that I might also be permitted to partake, I agreed that we should remain and keep watch on developments. Shortly the two men came back from the forest with several three-foot lengths of a vine about wrist-size in diameter but with no *yagé* leaves. The vine pieces were sent to a village across the river; there the brewing of the *ayahuasca* would start. Meanwhile the two men returned to the forest in search of the *yagé*. We waited around the *tambito* for a couple of hours hoping the men would return with the necessary leaves to complete the mixture of ingredients. Then Córdova mentioned his curiosity as to how the vine was being prepared and we took the launch across the Rio Tigre to the brewing village so that he could investigate. Córdova returned after a few minutes' visit in one of the houses and boarded the launch. Waving his arms and with an expression of disgust on his face he said, "We have been wasting our time. Let's go!"

As the launch got underway Córdova told me that the preparation of the *ayahuasca* which he saw was completely inadequate. The boiling down process was taking place in a dirty, old, beat-up aluminum pot watched over by a small boy. Taking such negligently prepared extract would result only in violent vomiting, acute abdominal cramps, and disorganized visions, if any. To obtain the desired results, Córdova said, the extract had to be prepared with extreme care and reverence in a special earthenware pot never used for anything else.

During the intervening years since our encounter on the Rio Tigre, working in the forest and conversing around our jungle campfires, I have come of course to recognize the authority with which Don Manuel spoke when he judged the negligent preparation of *ayahuasca* at Santa Elena. The basis for his understanding of the obscure medicinal properties of plants became apparent. And from small daily incidents in our months together, gradually I became aware of the scope of knowledge and depth of commitment Córdova brought to his efforts. He was totally involved in the alleviation of human suffering. The deeper I probed, however, the more I sensed his frustration. His attempts to perpetuate and hand down his rare knowledge had thus far failed. Healing people gave him great satisfaction. But for a master it was not enough. Implicit in his indoctrination into the secrets of *ayahuasca* and the knowledge of a *curandero* (healer) was an obligation to pass on the esoteric learning by training someone in turn to carry it on. Since this knowledge, apparently, was derived from a source no longer in existence, his failure added an urgent poignancy to Don Manuel's account of his own life. And so I became his chronicler and found myself under the spell of his tales of "non-ordinary reality." I saw that my position in the Amazon was not only to chart landscapes but to gather the shards of an esoteric teaching. I had been enlisted in the service of the same ancient lineage that had kidnapped and trained Córdova.

During our sojourn on the Rio Tigre I began to sense, with Córdova's help, the nuances of what river people expect from their daily existence in this region of the upper Amazon. My understanding came from our encounters like the one with those two Indians preparing the batch of *ayahuasca* at Santa Elena. These incidents gave me a feeling for the milieu in which Manuel Córdova had learned, tested, and now practiced his art of diagnosis and healing.

From Santa Elena, Córdova and I went down the Rio Tigre to the mouth of its largest tributary, the Rio Corrientes, and then up this meandering stream to Copalyacu. At a fork in the river where Copalyacu Creek flows into the Corrientes we came to a small village of three or four palm-thatched houses. We pulled up to the high bank where two men were working on an overturned canoe, attaching a small keel. One of them, we found out later, was a Jívaro Indian,[4] Bautista Mucushua, who by some now-obscure quirk of fate had been left as a small child here on the Rio Corrientes, far from the tribal territory of his people living in Ecuador.

We asked Mucushua if he could suggest someone with knowledge of the local geography and forests to act as our guide for the area. He suggested his son, Umberto. We talked to the young man, and he joined our party on board the launch for a few days. First, after consulting with Umberto, we decided to examine the forest up Copalyacu Creek. Entering the creek, Umberto pointed out to us the location of an abandoned Murato Indian[5] village. Then he recounted the story of how a group of these Indians had gone down the Corrientes a short ways on a mission of vengeance to the home of José Rios who traded with them. It seemed that the Muratos blamed Rios for the death of one of their children, saying that he killed the child with his witchcraft.

Knowing that their *patrón*, Rios, bathed late every afternoon on a small raft at the riverbank in front of his house, these Muratos hatched a plan. From their camp they came floating downriver in a big canoe with a paddle-man in each end of the craft guiding its progress. Several others, however, were hidden under banana leaves in the bottom of the canoe. In the late afternoon, just as they had planned, these Indians found José Rios bathing on the balsa raft at the river edge below his house which perched high on the riverbank. As the canoe came alongside the raft a tapped signal on the gunwale brought the hidden Indians up from under the banana leaves with their bows and arrows at the ready. A few silent paddle strokes and the canoe veered away, returning upstream, leaving Rios bleeding to death from the barrage of arrows suddenly launched against him from a distance of only a few feet.

After this, Umberto told us, the Muratos all disappeared into the forest before any authorities could investigate. The nearest source of help consisted of the army post at Sargento Lores two days travel downriver at the mouth of the Rio Corrientes. Córdova, as his contribution to the story, explained to me that the Muratos were notorious for being difficult to deal with. He said they would kill and rob on the Rio Pastaza and then disappear overland to the small headwaters of the Rio Tigre or Corrientes. There, as soon as enough time had passed so that they could safely return, the Muratos planned and executed a new atrocity and moved back to the Pastaza.

Umberto told us that a group of Murato families had a camp now on Shimbillo Creek a few hours' travel above Copalyacu. We went up Copalyacu Creek in our launch, making several stops on the way to examine the forest. When we came to the mouth of the Shimbillo Umberto agreed to lead us up to the Murato camp in our canoe with outboard motor. Although we started early in the morning, it took us more than half a day to reach the Muratos in their small jungle clearing on the bank of the stream. The last few miles we had to navigate through overhanging vegetation that completely covered the small stream. When we arrived mid-afternoon, there was only one man in the village with the women and children, a young Indian with shoulder-length hair. *Chukuchasapa*, Córdova called him after we left. It means long-haired witch doctor. Only the medicine man or shaman lets his hair grow long among the Muratos. We stayed there just long enough to take some pictures, for which Córdova first asked permission in their language, a variant of Quechua. On our return downstream we saw at a sharp turn in the creek the Murato men rolling cedar logs into the river to make up a raft for trading further downriver. We didn't stop but waved and shouted a greeting as the swift current carried us by quickly. Umberto told us that this was not the group of Muratos which had killed José Rios.

On our arrival back at Copalyacu the next day, Bautista Mucushua questioned us at length about how his son had performed as our guide. He seemed pleased when we told him we were well satisfied. He told us that he had given lots of time and attention to trying to make the boy responsible.

After returning from the Shimbillo and Copalyacu Creek excursions, we spent two days in the forest up the Corrientes above Copalyacu village. As we returned on our way back down the Corrientes to the Rio Tigre we stopped at Copalyacu to leave and pay off Umberto, our guide. Having an interest in the Jívaro Indian tribe, I thought of asking Bautista Mucushua about his people and the circumstances of his being left at Copalyacu. Inquiring for him I was told that he had gone downriver to the Rios place, which was now occupied by a son, Rafael, and his wife.

Out of curiosity about the place where José Rios had been assassinated by the Muratos and a desire to talk again with Mucushua, I suggested we stop at the Rios farm on our way down the Corrientes. We climbed the steps dug in the steep clay bank up to the house and we found Mucushua and young Rios well into a drinking bout. They were guzzling home-made cassava beer. The wife brought Córdova a large bowl full to the brim. He tried it and pronounced it good.

The two neighbors stood around talking in a fairly incoherent language full of *carajos, putas,* and similar vulgar terms. It didn't seem like a situation which would yield any useful information, nor a discussion to which we could contribute, so we excused ourselves and went our way on down the Corrientes to the Rio Tigre.

A few days later we came out at the mouth of the Tigre on the Rio Marañon. It was the weekend and we decided to stop to discuss our forest explorations with an old friend of Córdova's, one Juan Peña-Herrera, who lived there at the mouth of the Tigre. Long conversations ensued about where the best forests of the region were located and what kind of timber was found where. When the subject changed to that of medicinal plants and their use, Peña Herrera asked Don Manuel abruptly, "Do you believe in witchcraft?"

Córdova replied, "That all depends on the circumstances, and by the way, what exactly do you mean—do I believe in witchcraft?"

"I will give you an example," responded our host. "During the war in 1943 I had men cutting wild rubber on the Rio Nahuapa where you have just been. One day I was dispatching a group of these men with their supplies into the forest, and at the same time trying to get ready to leave for Nauta[6] downriver where I buy my supplies. Just as I was about finished with the last of my men and was ready to leave, I had a very painful spasm in my back that almost bent me double. Finally with the help of my wife I was able to get into the canoe and go down to Nauta, but I was in great pain all the way. At Nauta I was barely able to get around town to the supply houses to buy the things I required. Several days later I returned home, still bent and in pain.

"When I got back here José Rios had just arrived from his place at the mouth of the Copalyacu on the Rio Corrientes. When he asked me what was the matter I explained to him how the pain in my back had started.

"Rios said, 'We will have to get to the bottom of this. Bring me a twist of tobacco and your can of creolin.'

"He then cut a piece of tobacco and chopped it up into small bits. These he put into a cup of water. The water soon turned dark brown and Rios poured some out into his cupped hand. Then he said, 'We will get to the bottom of your trouble now. I am going into a trance.' He poured the tobacco juice into the right nostril of his nose. Then he poured out creolin into his left hand and took this into his left nostril. And then he fell to the floor in a trance.

"When Rios woke up after a half an hour or so he seemed dazed for a while, and didn't say anything. Later he ate some food and told me, 'Look, Ramírez down the river wanted to marry your wife and you took her away from him. He has asked some *brujo*, some witch, to put the hex on you. That is the reason for your back trouble. But never mind. I can take care of them. In a day or two your trouble will disappear.'

"And it did, too!" Peña-Herrera said to us. "So that is what I mean, Córdova, when I ask if you believe in witchcraft. In a day my back trouble went away completely. What do you think of that?"

Don Manuel was silent for a moment with some inward thought, and then he asked, "Was that José Rios-Rios from up on the Rio Ucayali?"

"Sure," replied Peña-Herrera, "but he had been living up on

the Corrientes near the mouth of the Copalyacu for several years. It was only a couple of years ago that the Murato Indians whom he traded with killed him for practicing witchcraft on them. They said he caused one of their children to die.''

Don Manuel shook his head. ''All that José Rios knew of witchcraft he learned from me. He was from my mother's family and came to live with us at Águano Isla when he became an orphan. But his knowledge was only superficial. That is why he got into trouble. The practice of witchcraft nearly always ends with someone being assassinated for revenge. Another perfect example is that of my old friend Chief Santos of the Secoyas up on the Rio Napo. When a woman died in a rival village they were sure Santos had killed her by witchcraft. And their only recourse was to assassinate Chief Santos, since their own witchcraft was not strong enough to kill him. I tell you, there are better ways of handling a problem such as curing your backache without using witchcraft, and as a matter of fact your backache probably cleared up of itself.''

Peña-Herrera tried to extend the discussion, but Don Manuel firmly changed the subject and refused to be led back into it. Peña-Herrera then launched into a long story about his experiences fighting the Ecuadorians while he was a sergeant in the Peruvian Army, stationed at the frontier border posts of Rocafuerte and Pantoja on the Rio Napo. In this area the border between Peru and Ecuador had been under dispute for centuries, and these are primitive Amazon forest outposts. When our host told us about how the insults traded back and forth across the present border had finally boiled up into a skirmish and how he became wounded, with his platoon on the point of retreat, he pointed at his wife. ''She was watching and rushed in, not to help me but to grab my gun and rally the troops.'' At this point in the story Rosa Panduro de Peña-Herrera, listening to her husband's tale, brought out an elaborate Army Certificate of Citation giving her credit for heroic bravery defending the fatherland in the battle against the ''ecuachos'' as Juan called them. Here at the mouth of the Rio Tigre there existed no cinema, television, hi-fi nor radio. Therefore the quality of one's hospitality depended on the interest stimulated by the conversation. Córdova and I have often, since that time, spoken of our animated visit with Juan Peña-Herrera and Doña Rosa.

When we finished cruising the forests on the Rio Tigre and its tributaries and left Peña-Herrera's place there at the mouth of the Tigre, we examined the timber up several of the smaller streams flowing into the Rio Marañon. One day cruising a prime timber boundary on the Rio Nahuapa we traversed an upland forest of tremendous mixed tropical hardwood trees—the habitat of cedar,[7] mahogany,[8] *aguanilla,*[9] *pashaco,*[10] *catahua,*[11] and many other species of impressive size. In this forest the upper tree canopy was so dense that little sunlight reached the ground to stimulate an undergrowth that might have impeded our passage. I noticed the great difference when we came to a large patch of jungle made up of small, misshapen trees all of one kind. The contrast was so striking that I stopped and asked Don Manuel about the cause. The small reddish-brown trunks supported only a few branches with a sparse crown of leaves. The completely barren ground heightened the contrast with the surrounding forest.

Córdova answered me without hesitation. "*Supai chacra*—devil's garden! Around these devil trees (*supai chacra caspi*)[12] nothing else will grow. Look, not even an ant on the ground, and the forest around a dead silence. *Que curiosidad*, the hold this small tree has on the rest of the forest. Remind me to tell you about the poisoned Rio Javarí. This is the tree the Remo Indians used to poison streams and thus keep out the invading rubber cutters."

We also checked the timber on the Rio Choroyacu, a narrow, blackwater stream which drained a large area of seasonal swamp. After the evening meal one day we were sitting on deck talking when Córdova said, "Here we should hear the swamp frog that has learned to talk English." And a few minutes later he put up a hand to stop our conversation. Off in the swamp there was indeed a frog croaking, with a sound that easily fit the expression "all right—yes, all right—yes," and Córdova exploded in laughter over the frogs which had learned to speak English.

Another evening on this same river we were trying to converse over the cacophony of what seemed like the raucous croaking of at least a million frogs nearby. And I said to Don Manuel, "Good Lord, how are we going to sleep tonight with all that racket going on?''

''Don't worry,'' he replied, ''it will stop in a few minutes.'' Barely were these words out of Córdova's mouth when, as if by his signal, every croaking frog stopped at the same instant, leaving us with ringing ears in a dead silence. Again my friend broke out in laughter. ''You see? Just like I said,'' Gradually then our hearing adjusted to the more delicate and varied sounds of the swamp forest—the plop of a tree fruit falling into the black water, the hum of an insect or the call of a night bird.

The intensity of my interest and involvement in all the other aspects and major events of Córdova's life grew with continued awareness of his total rapport with the Amazon jungle. Each new incident whether it concerned an explanation of the mores of some isolated Indian tribe, the singing behavior of swamp frogs, or a discussion of the effects from taking *ayahuasca* added wonder and new mystery to my exploration of the Rio Tigre and beyond.

4

Winged Death

On one of my later trips to Peru I found Córdova in Lima, visiting family who lived there in the capitol. We spent several days together in Miraflores, a residential suburb of the city. At this time I was especially interested in obtaining information on specific cases of serious illness that Don Manuel had treated successfully. We were seated together on a comfortable bench in a small park adjacent to a busy thoroughfare taking the air one afternoon when Don Manuel reached behind us to pick a leaf off a tall shrub shading our resting place. "Hmm," he mused, examining carefully both sides of it. "From this plant I could make an effective potion to cause abortion."

Another day we were people-watching from the same location when Córdova let a long whistling sigh escape his pursed lips. I looked at him and he pointed to a pair of attractive young ladies walking along the sidewalk. "See those girls?" he asked. "Reminds me of my youth. That pretty little plump one looks just like Nieves when I stole her from the padres at Requena and took her upriver to my forest camp. A beautiful girl, she was, and full of life, too!"

Later, during a discussion of the circumstances of his escape from his Indian captors, he said to me, "*Amigo* Lamb, if conditions had been different I might have stayed on in the forest with those Indians for a long time. But the family ties of my early boyhood had been strong. And my ancestral background did not have its origin among forest-dwelling primitives of the Amazon, but came from those of the Iberian Peninsula. When my training with the use of the vision vine activated a clairvoyant channel that brought premonitions of tragedy and death at home I felt an irresistible impulse to escape somehow and return to my people. Beside that, I was aware of a concerted attempt on the part of our enemies there in the forest to assassinate me and thus eliminate the source of firearms from my group of Indians. And even if I had stayed, with the falling rubber prices arms were going to be more difficult to obtain in the future. I had visions of my bones rotting away unburied in the jungle. All these things made it impossible for me to stay."

And I asked him, "Didn't you find it difficult, after so many years, living as an Indian in the forest, to readjust to your former way of life? And all that jungle medicine you had learned about, how did you adapt that to the needs of civilized people?"

BOTH ADJUSTMENTS WERE GRADUAL, CÓRDOVA REPLIED. AT FIRST MY worst trouble was to learn to tolerate wearing clothes again. That really bothered me, though only for a short time. And soon I went right back in the forest; work in the forest was all I knew how to do. But I didn't return to the remote Huni Kui territory over there between the headwaters of the Rio Juruá and the Rio Purus. In fact I've never gone back there to this day.

When I escaped from my captors and returned to Iquitos it was about the end of the first World War in Europe. As a result of the war there came a temporary rise in rubber prices. This made it possible for me to find work soon after my return and I went back to the forest, working with rubber cutters. Most of these people were Indians of one tribe or another. So in essence I returned to the dangers and conflicts from which I had just escaped.

The tribal lives of the forest-dwelling Indians of the Amazon were subject to devastating pressures by the invading rubber exploiters seeking riches from rubber that could be extracted from the bark of various forest trees and then sold. Hostile tribes were forced into conflict by the invasion as they sought to escape and establish new tribal hunting territories in country already occupied by other tribes. In turn, the surviving Indians fought the invaders to avoid being enslaved as rubber cutters and to protect their women and children from abuse.

It was reaction to these very same pressures that resulted in my capture by the Huni Kui, whom some people call the Amahuaca. They worked out among themselves the strategy of capturing a young white man who could obtain firearms for them. This they hoped would give them a lasting defense against invasion. Some quirk of fate thrust me into this drama. What I learned about life in the forest living with the Huni Kui helped me protect myself after escape.

Within a few weeks after my return to Iquitos about 1917, I had a job as *matero*, rubber-tree finder, with Jorge Borda & Company. They had rubber-gathering camps in the Rio Tapiche area upriver from Iquitos, with headquarters at a place called Callao on the lower Tapiche. Borda sent me up the Rio Blanco, a tributary of the Tapiche, to reorganize the operations of Renaldo Yori. So you see I was right back in the forest. Yori was an Ecuadorian whom Borda had financed to organize rubber gathering operations for the company there on the Rio Blanco. When he came to this area, Yori had brought Witoto, Santa Rosa, and Cocama Indians to work for him out of a central camp at Zapallero. But with the fluctuating rubber prices Yori couldn't meet his obligations and went broke. I was assigned to take over his Indians and rubber-cutting trails in the forest.

There were six families of Witotos from the Rio Putumayo under Chief Segua; five families of Santa Rosas from Ecuador, called Mañanitas; and five families of Cocama Indians called Iraricas. Each group of families had its working area in the forest assigned, and came to Zapallero to turn in rubber for supplies. Nearby at the mouth of Capanahua Creek the French Padre, Enríque Nicole from the Mission at Requena, had a small chapel and worked there with groups of Mayo and Remo Indians. Padre Enríque was of great help to me in reorganizing Yori's operations. He understood the problems of working with Indians and keeping them satisfied.

During my first night in the good Padre's camp, sometime after midnight, my acute Indian-trained protective sense of any change in the surrounding forest picked up some nearly imperceptible sound and I roused from a light sleep. This sensitivity to my surroundings made it possible for me to exist in situations where others lost their lives. Now a scarcely discernible but persistent pulsation, which I could feel almost as much as hear, vibrated in the stillness of the jungle air. Not a leaf in the forest moved. Instantly alert, I tested the sound with every pore of my body as my hammock swayed slightly back and forth where it hung in a palm-thatched *tambito* in the forest. The direction of the sound was impossible to discern. It was only a slight pulsating throb that rose and faded.

Then nearby an answer came in a louder voice. The Inucuini[1] Indians, the jaguar people, were exchanging messages on the *dunduri,*[2] the big log drum. I had not yet, being a newcomer to this area, learned to read these pulsating Indian communications. I awakened the Padre from a sound sleep to determine the urgency of the now animated exchange being carried on the night air.

"Just time for the dry season gathering of these Remo Indians for a dance," he told me.

At that point there was no chance for further sleep, and the Padre stirred up the coals of the fire to make a pot of coffee. Savoring the sweet, black brew, Padre Enríque told me the story of how an Inucuini *curandero* (healer) had saved his life from jungle fevers.[3] In this same camp where we now talked he had been on the verge of death when the people brought him a bitter potion to drink. The fever, he said, went down almost as he drank and in a few days he was fully recovered.

Well, you can see, the jungle was still my life and I knew there was much more to learn from the forest and its people. But the unstable rubber market complicated our lives. Prices soon began to fall again. Traders going broke abandoned their trading posts in the forest, and the Indians they had supplied. In the process, adjustments and tensions of another kind developed as the invaders withdrew. The Rio Blanco country became especially dangerous as the abandoned groups of rubber-cutting Indians, on their own again, took the worst things learned from the retiring exploiters and combined that knowledge with skills drawn from the perennially brutal life of the forest.

Casa Borda was a well-organized company fighting for survival. In the predicament of an uncertain market the best solution seemed to be that of concentrating production efforts in areas where high volume rubber extraction was possible. Don Jorge Borda decided, because of my forest experience, to send me exploring for new forest areas with potential for *caucho* production.

Casa Borda was allied with Casa Morey which had the best fleet of motor launches operating in the Peruvian Amazon. After consultation between Jorga Borda and Felipe Morey, it was decided that I should explore the region between the village of Pebas on the Amazon below Iquitos and the Rio Putumayo to the north. If I found no good *caucho* forest there I was to continue on to investigate the Rio Javarí. Therefore I took the launch San Pablo of the Morey fleet from Callao on the Tapiche and went down the Amazon to Pebas. Here I explained to the Casa Morey trading agent that I was seeking highland *caucho*-type forest, and soon he had me off on my way to explore Tikuna Indian territory. The Tikunas preferred to live way back in the highlands at the headwaters of the small creeks in locations as far from the main rivers as they could find. Here in isolation they attempted to maintain their independence. They didn't exactly welcome visitors from the outside, as I found out soon enough.

By arrangement of the Casa Morey agent in Pebas I found myself in a small canoe with a silent Tikuna companion paddling up Ampiyacu Creek to the north. These Indians use a tiny canoe and a tremendous round-bladed paddle. The combination is well adapted to rapid travel in small streams. I sensed the faintest sign of recognition and approval from my reserved and reticent companion when, after a few strokes with my paddle, I could produce the same dry, crackling sound that he did as he pulled his paddle through the water at a certain angle. This sound comes from the tiny whirlpools playing around the paddle when efficient application of force against the water is made with one of these huge paddles.

As we navigated in and out of the overhanging vegetation of the creek bank I commented on the plants, birds, animals, on sounds, smells and signs that we encountered along the way. My silent companion began to respond when he realized that my knowledge of the forest and my ability to pick up its traces were as good or better than his. By the time we arrived at the first Tikuna village (several days back into the interior from the Amazon) my companion regarded me as an equal. He would not have to apologize to his tribesmen for bringing me into their territory.

On approach to the first riverbank settlement, Nino, my guide, began making a loud explosive sound with his paddle at each stroke. Alerting his friends to our arrival, he told me. Pulling up to the village landing we sat in the canoe at the creek bank fully an hour before making a move to disembark. Tikuna custom, according to Nino. He also told me that his people tested a newcomer's courage by their welcome encounter. "Don't flinch," he warned me.

Finally Nino shouted "We come!" Then, following his lead, with slow deliberate movements we stepped onto the shore and started up the bank. So far we had neither seen nor heard a single person. But as we entered the shadows of the first large palm-thatched house a phalanx of scowling men confronted us with raised spears.

One shouted, "You came? Where from? What for? Who be you?"

Nino pushed the spears aside as we walked through the group and turned to face them again. Then he explained in a few words who, why, and where from. In a few more minutes we were all drinking *masato*, fermented *yuca* beer, offered in large calabash bowls by the women. After this ceremonial drink normal conversation prevailed until all felt their curiosity satisfied.

Later I found out that the Tikunas lived then in several isolated, extended-family villages scattered in the forest throughout the highlands, between the headwaters of Ampiyacu, Algodon and Cotuhe Rivers. There was little interchange or traffic between these villages. However, as I traveled around among them exploring the forest of the region for *caucho*, my reputation as a man of the forest always seemed to precede my arrival at a new village. The jungle telegraph worked well in Tikuna territory. In recent years I heard that the Tikunas have moved to more isolated country in nearby Brazil.

My hunt for *caucho* in Tikuna country was a failure because the tree did not grow in that forest. But in trading jungle lore with these Indians I soon found out about *ampihuasca*, the poison vine from which *curare* extract is made. The Tikuna, you know, are famous, even in parts of the Amazon Valley distant from their territory, for producing the best quality *curare* available anywhere for use on poisoned arrows and blowgun darts.

The plants they used were new to me because they did not appear in the forests where I had traveled south of the Amazon. I was interested in learning the details of the extraction process, but found it a carefully guarded secret between a few select men of the tribe. Each one handed it down to one carefully selected male relative within his close family group. From generations of experience they were convinced that not everyone could withstand the strong ritual magic required to control the proper blending of the poisonous ingredients in the tediously slow boiling-down process.

Finally, from comparing notes on our knowledge of the jaguars and other forest cats, I got close to old Chief Izidoro of the Jaguar Clan. His village was called Place-of-the-Soaring-Swallows. One day when we were talking alone together in the forest I convinced him that I could turn myself into a black jaguar with the magic of *ayahuasca*. Izidoro admitted that he knew of the effects of this vine, which he called *cipó caapi*. He took the extract while getting ready to make a batch of *curare*. We agreed to exchange secrets. I would show him how to turn himself into a black jaguar, most feared and astute beast of the forest. He would show me the magic of making *curare*. Then together we went into the forest to gather the plants we needed.

First Izidoro took me to his secret place in the forest where he brewed, as he called it, the winged death. As we came into the tiny clearing in the forest undergrowth beside a small clear stream, something strange about the place caused me to pause and look around carefully. It was shadowy dark under the canopy of a group of large buttressed trees. Grotesquely twisted lianas hung from high branches and a wind rattled leaves in the treetops a hundred and fifty feet above our heads but did not penetrate to the ground. The trees groaned softly from the wind pressure, and far off in the treetops out of sight the call of a large billed toucan reminded us of other life in the forest. Izidoro started cleaning up the few dead leaves and branches that had accumulated on the ground since he had last used the place. After my moment of testing the feel of the surroundings I helped with the clean-up. Then we cut palm leaves and small poles with which to make a small lean-to shelter. After this it took us two days to gather the firewood and plants required for our magical preparations. Izidoro examined the plants with meticulous care and selected only those parts with appropriate qualities.

Ampihuasca is a large woody vine that hangs down from the tree tops where its leaves compete with the big trees for sunlight. The vine uses tree branches for support. We found a place where several stems were draped in large loops and twisting turns traversing downward from the tree branches over a hundred feet above us. Izidoro carefully examined them and selected one. Compared to the others it had a medium diameter, some four inches, a fairly straight stem in which my companion pointed out the abundance of irregularly spaced, deep indentations.

Grasping the selected vine by hand and foot, Izidoro climbed up into the tree tops. There he cut it loose. It came crashing to the ground, as he descended by another vine. We cut the selected vine into three-foot lengths, made bundles of the sections, and carried them back to our small clearing in the forest. Before tying up the bundles for carrying, Izidoro showed me how we should strike every piece several times against a tree trunk to dislodge the scorpions that might be hiding in the indentations of the vine stem. Mother-of-the-scorpion, they consider *ampihuasca*, and believe that between the two life-forms they brew their joint poisons. Beating our vine segments on the trees we dislodged several scorpions. Two of these Izidoro captured with a pair of twigs and placed in a small covered calabash. They would be added to the boiling mixture near the end to add their spirit and poison to the *curare* extract.

Leaving our bundles of *ampihuasca* at the clearing we went a long distance to a swampy place. There, beside a blackwater pool, we found a small tree two inches in diameter with the markings of a boa skin on its trunk. We dug up several long roots of this tree and carried them back. Near our camp we gathered selected leaves from two different low shrubs. In our supplies from the village we had brought out special cooking pots, several green tobacco leaves, and a small basket of fresh, tiny, red-hot peppers—*pucuna urco*,

Izidoro called them.

When all these were arranged in our cool dark spot in the forest in orderly fashion to Izidoro's satisfaction, he carefully reviewed each plant and went over it by name. Then it was time to start looking for *cipó caapi*, my *ayahuasca*. All this while we had been on a sparse diet of unsalted roast jungle partridge and boiled white *yuca* (cassava). Now on the last day we fasted, ate nothing at all.

Izidoro said that *cipó caapi* held the strongest, most dangerous spirit of the forest, and its force would lead us to the right place to find our soul-vine. After we followed this spirit to its chosen site, we chanted incantations to the liana in our different tongues, Tikuna and Huni Kui. And then we cut several pieces to take back with us to our secret forest camp.

In talking over the extraction of *ayahuasca* with Izidoro I found out that there were no *chacruna* or *yagé* plants in this forest from which to get the leaves I had always used in the mixture. He told me that they made a cold-water extract by soaking the mashed vine in water, rather than boiling as I was accustomed. Knowing that a plant species can vary from one location to another I decided to go along with the local method of preparing *cipó caapi* extract. While we pounded the vine and put it to soak in a large clay pot I told Izidoro to think only about the black jaguar and the things he wanted to learn from the animal. Again we chanted, each in his own language. Long since we had discarded all our clothing except for the *taparabo*, tail cover, and had become true creatures of the forest.

At dusk we poured off the greenish-brown liquid and strained it through a piece of bark cloth. From a small round calabash cup each of us drank down his bitter potion. I knew it was weaker than my boiled preparation when my companion insisted we must drink a second cupful to assure a good effect.

Then we sat down in our hammocks and waited. I told Izidoro to let me sing. When the vine took over he would understand. Closely in the flickering light of our fire I watched, and when I saw a shudder pass through the body of my companion I knew it was time to start the jaguar chants and sounds.

Imitating all the jaguar sounds my Indian captors had taught me, interspersed with precise songs and chants, I brought the black jaguar into our visions. He transfixed us with his flashing yellow eyes. Gradually Izidoro seemed to blend with the body of the black cat. They wandered off into the forest as one and I followed in my dreams. Even if I could describe them adequately, that big cat showed my Tikuna friend things you would not believe—how the poisonous snakes produce their venom and what plants to chew for recovery from an accidental, potentially fatal encounter; also why the giant boa has no poisonous fangs and how to avoid its stupifying breath and bone-crushing embrace. Trained to think as an Indian, I took myself back to those native modes of thought, bearing my companion along on a strange journey.

In the morning, while the mist still drifted through the tree tops, we awoke from our dreams, built up the fire, then washed the bitter taste from our mouths. Each chewing a piece of sugar cane, we talked about what we had seen in our visions and began preparation of the extract that flies with the arrow and dart to bring its victims the winged death.

The round large-bottomed pots we rubbed inside with special crushed green leaves to make them leak-proof and then we placed them over a bed of hot coals to dry. Izidoro again took each plant ingredient in his hands and spoke its name. Then we mashed the *ampihuasca* by pounding it on a stone with a heavy wooden club, being careful not to lose a splinter of vine or a drop of its juice. With the pots dry and warm over the fire we added water from the creek and put in the tied-up small bundles of the mashed vine.

Then we scraped the roots of the boa plant. The vapor from this burned our eyes. These scrapings Izidoro put in a leaf funnel; then he filtered water through them into the cooking pot. From a tree nearby a caustic latex was extracted and added—then tobacco leaves, the fiery hot peppers, leaves from the bush-which-talks-to-the-wind, and later the two scorpions from the calabash cage. All this we did with the greatest care and deliberation, naming each ingredient as it was added to the mixture. The slightest misstep from traditional ways could spoil the whole process.

This mixture Izidoro kept at a low simmer with appropriate incantations all the first day and night. The second morning we poured off the brownish liquid into a clean pot through a filter of tree-bark cloth. Then this simmered all day and all night. The washed-out ingredients we scattered in the forest so they could not be identified by anyone and thus give up their magic.

On the third morning the finishing process started. The coffee-colored liquid Izidoro decanted off into a smaller pot to remove any sediment. A slight foam began to form on the surface as the simmering continued. These suds he skimmed off; then he dipped several darts into them. He dried these over the hot coals. Then we went to the creek. Earlier when we were bringing water to the pots, we had seen a big green toad along the stream. Now we found him again and pricked him with a poisoned dart on the soft white belly under his left hind leg. Putting him back on the ground again, we prodded him with a stick. When the toad could move no more after the fourth jump, Izidoro shouted "Ha!" in a loud voice, and smiled.

Back at the fire the most critical part of the *curare*-making was still to be carried out, but we knew from the toad test that the batch was good. Now my companion could not leave his brewing poison for a moment. With a hawk-wing fan and moving the hot coals around to obtain even distribution of heat, he watched and waited. A few bits of foam were removed, and he warned me again to be sure that I did not breathe the pleasantly fragrant vapors.

As we watched together a slight irridescent film formed on the surface of our liquid. Immediately Izidoro dipped a dart stem into the surface and lifted it. A long, thin stiff thread formed, and again my friend shouted "Ha! *La punta*—it's done!" With a single motion he scraped all the hot coals out from under the pot. And we ate some *yuca* and chewed sugar cane while the batch cooled. In a few minutes the winged death, about the consistency of honey, was dipped off carefully by Izidoro into small round calabash containers, each with a fitted lid.

The secret of *curare* was mine to use when needed and Izidoro could walk in the forest with the black jaguar to learn still more from him. Each of us had a new secret fixed in his mind and felt content with the result of the exacting five-day ordeal we had shared. Knowing how to make *curare* would prove valuable to me later, but now, having found no *caucho* in Tikuna country, I had to move on to the Rio Javarí to continue my exploration.

5

Poisoned Rio Javarí

MENTION OF THE RIO JAVARÍ ANYWHERE IN THE AMAZON VALLEY WILL bring a shudder of horror from your listeners. Padre Avencio[1] in his book *Asi Es La Selva* says "This river is the most sorrowfully celebrated in all of Amazonia." People dread the river because of the terrible jungle fevers that attack those who work or travel there. I myself was warned many times about the danger of Javarí fever before going there to explore for *caucho*, and, as a means of precaution, I resolved to find the source of this malady. The few people I had seen suffering from what was called Javarí fever did not seem to me to have *paludismo* (malaria) even though most people considered that to be the cause. On the Rio Galvez, a tributary of the Javarí, I found my answer.

There one day, working my way up a small stream called Remo Creek (named after the Indians who went by that name), I was carefully steering my canoe through the overhanging vegetation when somehow I sensed the presence of people nearby. Cautious not to be caught at a disadvantage in such an isolated spot, I slipped around a high bank and there came face to face with a group of naked Indians bathing in the stream. They were as surprised as I was, and for a moment all of us remained transfixed, held by each other's stares. Their faces and bodies were painted with the familiar patterns of my former companions of the forest, the Huni Kui. So I spoke to them—a greeting of friends—in the language of my Indian captors.

You could see the understanding and pleasure break out on their faces; still, the women and children slipped away like shadows after the first frozen moment. As the men spoke I found their language was somewhat different, but soon we had a flow of conversation and understanding going back and forth. I carefully observed all the niceties of the Huni Kui on meeting a distant tribesman, commenting on the condition of the forest at this time, its effect on game hunting. And gradually we came to more specific and immediate affairs—like where was I from and what was I doing? I parlayed by posing questions in return. The palaver ended by my being invited to their village, a cluster of small palm-thatched huts well back from the stream. Here one of the old women brought me a bowl of *masato* (fermented cassava) to drink and then served the headman.

As we talked and drank I explored their knowledge of the country for information I needed. According to them the *caucho* trees which I sought existed in abundance only on the highlands at the headwaters of the Rio Javarí where some of their tribesmen lived. They called themselves Inucuini; these are an offshoot of the same lineages as Huni Kui tribe, and their name means jaguar people. These were some of the same people that worked with Padre Enríque on the Rio Blanco where I had been recently.

I realized I would have to spend several days here in order to prepare a smooth departure. And one day while we were all bathing in the stream near their village I started to drink the water from my cupped hands. "No, no, no," they all said in unison, with raised hands and a look of great concern on their faces. "The water is poisoned," they told me. Then in explanation they took me to a nearby devil's garden—a patch of the *supai chacra* or devil's garden trees. There they demonstrated how they mashed up together the leaves, bark, and roots of this tree *(supai chacra caspi)*[2].

Those Remo Indians then put their oozing reddish mass of mashed plants into small woven baskets which they suspended out of sight at several places in the stream. They told me anyone drinking a few times from the stream below would die of terrible fever and pains—the Javarí fevers. Only this way, they said, could they keep the hated invading rubber cutters out of their territory. Then they showed me the plants to use and how to prepare an antidote, which no doubt had been given Padre Enríque to save his life on the Rio Blanco. Those Remo Indians also showed me how to prepare and use a remedy for snake bite and another for toothache from this devil's garden tree. It is a great secret of nature that many poisonous plants have medicinal properties if used properly. This is the way the world was created.

Among the Remo I saw for the first time that tiny monkey we call *leoncito*[3] (little lion) because its face resembles a miniature lion. This dwarfed animal, no bigger than my thumb, was riding on the ear of one of the children when I asked about it. In my hand it crawled around from finger to finger, a perfect child's pet, almost. In recent years animal exporters have found out about this curiosity from the Rio Javarí and have exported many to zoos and pet shops. But there is one drawback to carrying this minute monkey around in your shirt pocket, on your shoulder, or elsewhere—it is constantly urinating on your clothing!

After a few days, with careful planning, I was able to slip away unnoticed, thus avoiding any possible complications with my hosts. On a moonlit evening I silently pushed my canoe into Remo Creek and paddled downstream all that night and the next day before letting up to rest when I came out again on the Rio Galvez. From then on you may be sure I took the greatest care about the source of my drinking water. The Javarí had a well-earned reputation as a man-killer then, a fame that still exists today.

You remember the story we heard a few weeks ago about the Iquitos man who owned a sawmill on the Rio Javarí? Every time he went down there on an inspection trip he became ill and had to return to Iquitos. After several incidents of this illness, which occurred only on his visits to the sawmill on the Javarí, he became suspicious of his local manager, who was probably stealing him blind. By careful investigation the owner discovered that his manager was giving him poisoned Javarí water to drink at meals. Probably some local Indian cutting logs for the sawmill had shown the manager how to use *supai caspi* to poison his boss just enough to make him go back home to Iquitos. In the end of course he got fired for his dishonesty and intrigue. But you can see, the Javarí plays its time-honored tricks!

From the mouth of the tributary Rio Galvez I continued on up the extraordinarily tortuous, blackwater, slow-moving Rio Javarí, to a trading post called Bolognesi, owned by José Incarnacíon Rojas. Here the Chamicuro Indians worked for Rojas extracting rubber from the forest on both the Peruvian and Brazilian sides of the river. Early in the rubber boom these Indians had made Rojas wealthy. He built a huge whitewashed house on a high river bank, and from there sent his many children off to be educated in England as they reached, one by one, the proper age.

Rojas was a friend of my *patrón*, Jorge Borda, and when he found that I worked for Casa Borda nothing was too good for me. He insisted that I spend a few days with him, resting from my trip upriver and giving him the news of the outside world. Rojas told me about the forest in the highland drained by the headwaters of the Javarí, Blanco, and Tapiche Rivers. And he told me how to find an overland crossing between Yaquerana Creek, a tributary of the Javarí, and Hubuya creek of the Rio Tapiche headwaters. By making this crossing I could go down the Tapiche to Casa Borda's trading post at Callao without needlessly retracing the route I had come.

The forests of this highland, especially the part drained by the upper Tapiche, made a lasting impression on me. Here was the only place visited on my long trip where *caucho* trees were abundant. The forest reminded me of the country I had lived in with the Huni Kui. I had no trouble finding the *varadero* (overland crossing between rivers) described to me by Rojas at Bolognesi, and on my way down the Tapiche I made plans to return to this country of abundant game and magnificent forest.

Arriving at Callao after many months' absence, I found rubber prices still on the decline. Because of this, Casa Borda was pulling its traders out of the troubled Rio Blanco area which was fast becoming a no-man's land. Francisco Ribeiro de la Guardia and Roque Noriaga, both of whom had worked with the Mayo, Remo, and Marubo Indian tribes, now abandoned the rubber trade. The Indians went back to the forest. Word came to us that José Rojas had died at Bolognesi on the Javarí, not so very long after I visited him, and the Chamicuro Indians were abandoned, since his educated sons did not know how or want to continue in the failing rubber business.

As a result of my report on the abundance of *caucho* trees in the forest of the upper Tapiche and the deteriorating conditions among the inhabitants of the Rio Blanco, Borda decided that I should transfer my operations with the Witoto, Santa Rosa, and Cocama Indians to the Rio Tapiche, where I could work with Juan Hidalgo Mafaldo. By this time I was well-known in the fast-growing town of Requena at the mouth of the Rio Tapiche. Recognized as a man who managed money and people for Casa Borda, I carried some mark of importance. But traveling and living alone was becoming less and less attractive to me, and I had my eye on a cute girl, a student at the Padre's Convent School there at Requena. When I determined after a few clandestine meetings that there existed a strong bond of mutual attraction between us, I convinced Nieves Ochoa that she could live with me. Then I stole her from the Padres and took her with me to the upper Tapiche.

Going upriver in a flotilla of canoes with our companion Indians we made contact, as instructed by Borda, with Juan Hidalgo at the mouth of Humayta Creek. On the way Nieves informed me that Hidalgo was her uncle, and I wondered what complications this might cause. When we arrived and explained our mission, Juan Hidalgo suggested that we locate on the unoccupied section of the river above him. So, at a place we called *Tamishi Manchari* (Fearful Vine) because of a thorny vine found in the forest there, we made a clearing on the river bank and built a house. The Witotos found a place that suited them above us at the mouth of Bombo Creek. Rufino Segua and his people expressed their enthusiasm for the country right away. The Mañanita and Irarica families located below us on the Tapiche.

I could tell from the time of our arrival that Juan Hidalgo was worried about my competence to protect his sister's favorite daughter, Nieves, living as I was in the wilds of the upper Tapiche with Indians from various tribes. Spurred by his penetrating questions one day soon after we came, I told him about my life with the Indians he knew as Amahuaca. I could see his doubt fading as my story progressed. When I had finished he told me that during the time of my story Nieves' father had gone with a group of *caucheros* on a *correria* (chase) to Amahuaca country of the upper Rio Juruá to steal Indian children. None of them ever returned.

I at once made the connection between this and an incident among my people, the Huni Kui. You recall that I objected to old Chief Xumu when a group of our hunters came back with human flesh from a raid on *caucheros*. I explained all this to Juan Hidalgo.

What a strange world, that it should fall on me now to bring the word to my young wife, and eventually the rest of her family, about how her father had been captured and his flesh eaten by Indians with whom I was living at the time. But he participated in the raids *(correrias)* the Huni Kui had offered as bitter justification when I tried to stop them from attacking rubber camps. If I had to place blame, it would not be on the Indians. In desperate times people need to act in accordance with the actual circumstances and to answer the attacks of another culture with their own. In the jungle there was no substitute for faithful allies and brute means of self-protection.

Juan Hidalgo, before our coming to the Rio Tapiche, had organized the remnants of the Capanahua Indian tribe to work with him on the Humayta Creek. And there were other rubber cutters below him on the river. One such group, Bidar Ruíz and his two brothers, had a camp at the mouth of Hubuya Creek. These brothers did the actual work of cutting *caucho* and kept a group of Witoto Indians as bodyguards. One of these Witotos, called Charco, had trouble with the Capanahua Indians and killed one of them from Juan Hidalgo's group.

This brought to arms the whole camp of Capanahua on Humayta Creek. They threatened to wipe out the Ruíz brothers and their Witoto guards. Between us, Juan Hidalgo and I convinced the Capanahua that this would only bring bigger trouble. And I promised Chief Huanichi that the offending Witoto, Charco, would leave the country. I sent word to the Ruíz camp that Charco was being reported to the civil authorities at Callao. When Charco responded with threats to eliminate all the rubber cutters on the upper Tapiche but his own *patrón* it was time for action.

I armed myself, went to the Ruíz camp, and took Charco prisoner. Then with the help of my Witotos we transported him to Callao where the civil authorities ordered him to return to his own country, the Rio Putumayo.

While at Callao turning over that bandit Charco I heard about more trouble on the Rio Blanco. When old man Rojas died at Bolognesi his abandoned Chamicuro Indians went to the forest on the Brazilian side of the Rio Javarí. There they were taken over by some Brazilian criminals, Dario Montes and the Ferreiros brothers. Soon, because of their stealing and looting, those bandits were forced to move to the Peruvian side. There they took up with the Mayo, Remo, and Marubo Indians, previously abandoned by Ribeiro de la Guardia. These people then started making raids from their new camps on Choba Creek of the Javarí headwaters.

At that time Lióncio Lopez gathered rubber for Borda on Platanoyacu Creek of the Rio Blanco. His place was attacked by Indian bandits. They killed his cousin Bonifacio Sanchez, carrying away his wife and children. Lopez himself escaped. He had recognized Dario Montes and the Ferreiros who led the attack, and made an official declaration against the bandits at Callao as he was returning to Iquitos. This is when the Peruvian government established an Army Guard post at Callao, though it was ineffective.

Also about this time Pio Rojas from Moyobamba came to the Rio Blanco to cut *balata*[4] gum as an independent operator. He had a commercial trading license and established his post at the mouth of España Creek after Padre Enríque Nicole had been forced to leave. The first thing Rojas did was to make friends with the bandits and start supplying them with arms. Later Pio Rojas led an attack on the guard post at Callao, where he was captured, made a confession, and was executed. At this time Borda asked Juan Hidalgo Mafaldo to organize his Capanahua Indians and join forces with Enríque Uresti and his Campa Indians working below Requena to run the criminals out of the Rio Blanco area. The Capanahua and Campa both had a reputation for bravery. They organized a drive and forced the bandits to move out, but soon the renegades came back to Yaquerana Creek on the Rio Javarí near the Rio Blanco headwaters. Even today there is still trouble with raids from this area. No one will live on the east bank of the Rio Tapiche because of these bandits. The Army has tried to control them but only gets its patrols surrounded in the forest from where they have to radio for help. Reports of air support and bombing even appeared in the

New York papers.

Here Córdova interrupted his story to leaf through a file of papers until he came to a clipping which he handed me. It was a United Press International dispatch from Lima that had appeared in the *New York Herald Tribune* of March 16, 1964:

> **Lima**
>
> Peruvian Air Force B-26's flew strafing sorties yesterday against half-naked, poison-arrow-shooting Coquima tribesmen who have cut off an army patrol in the Amazon jungle near the Brazilian border.
>
> Air Force planes dropped grenades, ammunition and food to the beleaguered column of 65 jungle troopers for the third straight day. . . . The column was en route to the Javarí River, which forms the border along Brazil's northwestern hump, where a gunboat was waiting to evacuate it. . . . The patrol was turned back by the Indians from its mission to patrol the Brazilian border and chart a projected jungle road from Requena to the border.
>
> The B-26's were attempting to clear a path for the patrol which reported it was blocked in its effort to reach the river, an estimated 40 miles away, by around 300 Indians.
>
> Bombs, rockets and napalm were used against the Indians in "blind" air strikes through the tops of towering jungle trees Friday and Saturday. . . .

As I handed the clipping back, Córdova continued:

THE BANDITRY AND VIOLENCE IN THE JAVARÍ-RIO BLANCO COUNTRY finally became so bad, as you can see, that the local government men, in desperation, came to me recently and asked me to go there and help calm the situation. I thought about it and discussed it with the Governor, but the project fell through when I was refused a guarantee of support for my family if I failed to return. After all,

I knew very well that neither I nor anyone else could just walk into the forest and tame several groups of abused, wild Indians. It will be a long time before that country settles down, in spite of anything *los Padres Catolicos*[5] or *los Linguisticos del Instituto Linguistico* do to try to eliminate the conflicts.

6

The Capanahua

BY THE TIME WE MOVED TO THE UPPER TAPICHE IN 1919 THE CAPANAHUA Indians of that region had already been more or less pacified. But Juan Hidalgo was still the only one who could work with them. He made friends with their chief, Huanichi, learned their language and furnished them supplies in return for the rubber they produced.

Hidalgo told us of many violent incidents in the past history of these Indians. Years earlier they had killed eighteen rubber cutters in a battle on España Creek of the Rio Blanco. Trinchera, a rocky rapids in the Tapiche about halfway between our camp and Callao was the location of many wild battles in the past. Here the Capanahua made their last organized stand as a tribal group. They continued to ambush individual rubber cutters in the forest and steal their equipment until Juan Hidalgo, working with Huanichi, convinced them to stop.

The Capanahua accepted me, especially when I learned to talk with them quickly and they found that I knew the forest. Their language was similar to that of the Huni Kui. I cured some difficult illnesses among them, too. They believed that sickness was caused by witchcraft and evil spirits. Therefore in treating these people, along with the medicine I gave them, I also convinced them that the offending evil spirits were expelled, as part of the cure. If this required sleight-of-hand removal of thorns from their bodies I could do this too.

With many patients it helps them to get well if, along with the medical treatment, you give them an explanation they can understand of the cause for their condition. However, I would not explain the treatment given to a superstitious forest Indian in the same way as I would discuss medication given the Belgian Ambassador to Peru or the former President of my country, who have also been my patients. But, regardless of the explanation, the plant extracts used in treatment must be scrupulously correct to improve the patient's condition. I learned many things from the Capanahua. The profession of medicine is like that of music. You never stop learning and improving your technique.

One of Chief Huanichi's men was killed when a tree fell on him in the forest. This Indian's wife went into a complete depression when she heard about the accident; she refused to eat, talk, or even move. Huanichi showed me how he prepared a cure for this condition. On a nearby creek called the Pedernal (Flint) there was a rock formation of liver-colored, flint-like stone.[1] A small piece of this stone was heated in the fire and then put in a small vessel of water where it promptly shattered. After being allowed to steep for an hour or so, this liquid was poured off and, with persuasion, given the woman to drink. Within a few hours her abnormally depressed feelings were relieved and soon disappeared.

Since leaving the Tapiche I have many times used this mineral preparation to bring mentally disturbed patients back to a normal state. You might ask how these Indians had discovered such a cure. All I can tell you is that some of them are the most curious beasts in the forests. Their brains are as big as yours and mine, and they are in a situation to use them.

We were often invited to Capanahua celebrations. They had several each year—for a wedding or the sale of a big lot of rubber or some such thing. And it would all start when Chief Huanichi signalled the scattered groups in the forest to gather at his house. This was done by sending a message on the hollowed-out log drum, the *dunduri.* The weird sound of this instrument, played on late at night when every leaf of the forest remains still, will carry for miles through the jungle and be relayed even farther by other drummers. I learned to interpret the *dunduri* messages and thus usually knew what event brought the Capanahua together.

They painted up one another's bodies with weird, geometric designs, red and black colors made from *achiote*[2] and *huito*[3] extracts. When all were satisfied with the body paint the drinking and dances started, accompanied by drums, flutes, and singing. The women prepared several kinds of intoxicating fermented beverages. The men, before they were too drunk, had a dance or sham battle where opposing groups of them fought with large black palm-wood clubs and lances. This always stimulated a display of defensive skill and personal agility accompanied by the loud clatter of the striking clubs and wild shouts of the men. In these encounters it always seemed that someone surely would be killed, but no one received as much as a scratch. The Indian kids practiced this mock battle from the time they could wield a stick. When the accumulated food was all gone, these celebrations of singing and dancing invariably ended with a shouting, groaning, weeping melee of drunkenness which sounded fierce but in which no on really got hurt. After sobering up for a day or two they went back to work to obtain their life needs from the forest. From Chief Huanichi I learned of a remedy for alcoholic intoxication and its after effects. Since leaving life in the forest I have found it useful also in curing cases of alcoholism and its complications.

The Capanahuas were good hunters. Sometimes they used dogs to assist in finding game. I remember one time when I was out hunting with Chief Huanichi. He had brought along his favorite hunting dog, *Chocoláte.* Off in the forest, several hours from camp, we came on a large band of *huangana,*[4] wild pigs. There were over a hundred in the *manada*, and we unlimbered our rifles at the first sight of stragglers. One of the pigs was only wounded and it started squealing and screaming. Instantly and with a loud clicking of tusks we were surrounded by the whole infuriated band and each of us had to take immediately to the nearest tree we could climb. But there was no place for *Chocoláte* to go nor time for him to run away.

We stayed up in the trees for several hours before that herd of *huangana* wandered off. The heat and stench of those wild pigs milling around our refuge trees clicking their teeth, waiting for us to come down or fall down, was nearly unbearable. When they had gone and we did come down we could find not a trace of *Chocoláte*, not even a brown hair. And we would have disappeared in the same way if we hadn't climbed up the trees out of reach.

The Capanahua had been feuding with the Remo Indians over

territory as long as any of them could remember. When the invasion of rubber cutters first began, the Capanahua had occupied a large territory from the Rio Juruá to the headwaters of the Javarí, including the Rio Blanco and the Rio Moa. Battling with both the rubber cutters and the Remo had reduced them to only a few families living on the upper Tapiche at Capanahua Creek and nearby. Later, after we left this country, Chief Huanichi moved the remnants of his people farther west to Ubuya Creek where what is left of the tribe now lives. This move was made in response to pressure from the Remo or Inucuini people. The Capanahua have now nearly disappeared as an organized and distinct group or tribe.

Several times small groups of Remo Indians visited us at our home, Tamichi Manchari, on the Rio Tapiche. These shy, secretive people remembered friendly contacts which I had made with them when I had worked in their territory on the Rio Blanco. They respected my knowledge of the forest. And we had long discussions about the curative properties of the forest plants.

I learned about *chicuro piripiri*[5] from these Remo Indians. A mixture of tobacco juice and the extract from the bulbous root of a small forest plant are the ingredients. According to them drinking this mixture on a calm night, isolated in the deep solitude of the forest, produces a reaction similar to that of taking *ayahuasca* (*honi zuma* in their language) under like circumstances. Both require a long period of preparation and fasting. They told me that many people could not overcome the nauseous reaction to taking *chicuro piripiri.* The man that did reach the stage of complete control they considered to be a great seer, a healer who could penetrate the many secrets of the forest. They also claimed that *chicuro piripiri* enabled one to see inside the body of a sick person and to determine the source of an illness. I never took it with them since I could do the same with *ayahuasca*.

While we were living on the upper Tapiche I made two rather long jungle trips. Casa Borda wanted me to explore the country south of the Rio Tapiche headwaters to see if I could find anything of value that we could extract from the forest. The rubber market continued to decline and new forest products were needed to sustain commerce in this undeveloped forest region. The country to the south of us was not an area with which Huanichi and his Capanahua were familiar, so I decided to take Rufino Segua and his Witotos with me to see what I could find. These Witotos came from the Rio Caraparana, a tributary of the Rio Putumayo, early in the rubber-boom days. They were among the best-adapted forest people I have worked with and even though this was new country for them I had confidence we could find our way back through this trackless and uninhabited country.

Rufino chose four of his young men and we all prepared personal equipment for a long pack trip overland. Since each person had to carry his own supplies, we limited ourselves to the essentials. I carried a 44 Winchester Repeater and the Witotos took 20-gauge shotguns. In addition to ammunition each of us carried a change of clothing, a string hammock, a machete, a little salt, and a few other small items of personal importance. We expected to live for several weeks entirely off the forest. This was nothing new to any of us. We all knew the fruit trees and shrubs, the ground roots and bulbs, and all the birds and animals we were likely to encounter that were good to eat.

On the first day out I saw Rufino gathering leaves from a bush and asked him why. He said it was of the same family as the *coca* plant his people on the Rio Putumayo used to chew to avoid fatigue on long trips. They had found this plant served the same purpose and he thought we would need it on our journey. I agreed with him and we used it regularly to good effect.

Game was plentiful in this forest and we had no trouble getting the food we needed. We ate only twice a day—at daylight before we started off and late in the afternoon when we stopped to make camp. We all knew by instinct how to keep our general direction even in the densest forest and on the cloudiest day. When we contacted game by sign or sound one of the boys would go after it and the rest of us would continue on. Depending on the length of the chase, the hunter would either intersect our route as we traveled or come into our camp in the evening loaded with prey that might include small forest deer, wild pig, tapir, agouti, partridge, wild turkey, and many other animals and birds.

Only twice on this trip of several weeks did we come upon signs of other people. When we were out about a week we came upon a petroleum exploration camp. They were examining the geology of the country between Contamana on the Rio Ucayali and the Brazilian border. In this camp I found a friend from Iquitos, engineer José Angúlo Rodríguez. He introduced me to the American geologist Dr. Harvey Bassler[6] who was in charge of the exploration. Here we traded game for supplies and asked them to leave for us a hidden cache to be used on our return trip. The camp was going to be abandoned anyway in a few days when they would be returning to Contamana.

At this stopping place Angúlo took me off into the forest to show me something he said would be of interest to me. We had walked maybe half an hour when I began to sense the putrid smell of a dead animal and my friend put a handkerchief over his nose. In a few more minutes we came on a place where all the jungle undergrowth had been torn up. In the middle of this lay the remains of a giant boa, the *yacumama*[7]. It was so foul we could not examine it closely. Angúlo told me that they had come on it in their explorations and had killed it over a week before. Dr. Bassler had asked his men to remove several hundred of the two-inch scales from its skin and cut out several vertebrae. These had been taken to Contamana for shipment to North America or Germany. I could not verify the size of the snake because of the smell, but Angúlo told me that the animal had been somewhat less than a meter (three feet) in diameter and more than fifteen meters (forty-five feet) in length. He told me he expected that Dr. Bassler would publish a description that would put an end to all speculation about whether or not the giant boa, the *yacumama,* really existed in the Amazon forest.

Angúlo said they had been very careful to shoot the boa from behind the head and then get out of the way. It is a common belief where these boas are found that the breath of the reptile kills its victims, that they capture their food by lying quietly in the forest and blowing their breath on any animal that goes by. Because of the precautions they had taken, Angúlo said, none of his group had yet suffered from this poisonous breath.

We left the boa camp as the geologists were getting ready to leave for Contamana, and we continued south through the forest for another week or more. One day we came upon a group of men cutting timber along a small creek. We asked them about their location and where they expected to take the logs out. They said the creek would carry the logs into the Rio Tamaya and that the cedar they were cutting was contracted to a sawmill at Pucallpa. Now we knew where we were and we decided to go back home. Again we traded fresh game for supplies and started out, this time retracing our route. On the way we picked up our supplies at the petroleum exploration camp, and arrived back home at Tamishi Manchari on the Rio Tapiche about a month after leaving.

We had not really found much but trees: petroleum was beyond the field of my knowledge. It was a rich and varied forest, but at that time there seemed to be nothing in it that could be exploited commercially. Today it is about the same except for a few valuable lumber species like cedar and mahogany that are being cut. My friend Angúlo and his oil geologist companions must have found good indications of oil though, because the El Oriente oil field is now located about where I ran into their camp.

With the price of rubber declining to the point where it became unprofitable to produce under wild forest conditions and with the hides of game animals, wild pig and deer, the only source of cash income, it began to look as though we would be forced to leave our forest home on the Rio Tapiche. Before doing this I decided to make a trip across the Brazilian border to Cruzeiro do Sul on the Rio Juruá. I wanted to check the rubber market in Brazil.

I took four men with axes and machetes and we went in two small canoes up the Tapiche past Bombo and Bombillo Creeks, as far as we could go, dragging our canoes through several rapids in the stream. When we had forced our way as far as possible by stream we hid the canoes and walked overland by a faint trail to the southeast. After about an hour we found, on a hilltop, a survey marker that fixes the border between Peru and Brazil. From here it was only two more hours' walk to a creek called Igarape Ramon that flows into the Rio Moa.

On the Igarape Ramon we made camp and started looking for a *paxiuba* palm suitable for making a canoe. We found a perfect big one, chopped it down, opened one side of the trunk, and then dug out the soft inner fiber leaving the hard outer shell. This made a good temporary water craft. The next day I sent all but one man back to the Tapiche with instructions to use one canoe, leaving the second for us, and to return to their homes near Tamishi Manchari.

My companion and I took our paddles—brought overland with us—along with a few supplies, shotgun and rifle, and embarked in our new canoe for the trip down the Rio Moa. After a couple of days' easy travel downriver we came to Valparaiso. This was a settlement of a few houses on the south riverbank near the mouth of Azul Creek. Here I hired a man named Oliveira, with a good, large canoe to take us downriver.

In about a week we arrived at the *fazenda* (the ranch) of Colonel Alfredo Mancio Lima located near the mouth of the Rio Moa. This was a big establishment at that time, several thousand acres of cleared land, the largest ranch in the Acre Territory of Brazil. On the river bank were a large house, a store, and a warehouse. We stopped at the store and when Don Alfredo heard that I had come over from Peru he invited me to stay at his home. He wanted to hear all the news from across the border.

In this isolated country without communications, anyone from outside was more than welcome for the news that he would bring. In those days, the 1920's, there was no radio, let alone television, in this isolated region. When Don Alfredo found that I could understand his Brazilian Portuguese and that he could pretty well make out my Spanish mixed with some Portuguese, we settled down for long hours of discussion and tales. He wanted to know all about Peru, and I had a few things to find out for myself. The market for rubber was as bad in Brazil as in Peru I soon learned. And it was here that I first heard about the destruction of the trading post on the Rio Purus from which I had escaped only a few years before when I had gone down the river by launch to Manaus and left my life in the forest with the Huni Kui.

The fragmentary reports which had reached Don Alfredo were to the effect that a large group of Indians with fantastic designs painted on their bodies had attacked the Purus trading post and completely destroyed it. I did not ask questions, but there was little doubt in my mind that these were the Indians I had lived with at Xanada,[8] up at the headwaters of the Rio de las Piedras.[9] I had often wondered about the aftermath of my escape from the Huni Kui. They must have thought that I had been captured, and for this had sought revenge. But I had not expected their reaction to be so violent.

Soon after my arrival at Mancio Lima's ranch, other men from trading posts up the Rios Juruá and Moa began to gather at Villa Mancio. Don Alfredo told me they were all going down the Rio Juruá to the town of Cruzeiro do Sul to organize a Masonic Lodge there. He invited me to come along and become a charter member.

A launch came up from Cruzeiro do Sul and transported us back down the river—a long tow of canoes out behind, transportation for our return upriver. It wasn't far and the trip took less than half a day. Cruzeiro do Sul was a good-sized town at that time, as big as Iquitos.

When we finally assembled in Mancio Lima's large house in the town, there were twenty-five or more men there, ready to join the Masonic Order. Don Alfredo and two or three others already belonged and from their manuals they instructed us in the secret and ancient methods of Masonic rituals and symbols. These teachings instilled in all of us a feeling of brotherhood, the obligation of charity to all men, and the requirement of adherence to established laws and customs. We were told that real privileges would come to us if we continued in the order and lived up to the intent of our instructions. The purposes of our lives would become clear, making it possible to avoid the gloom and stress of error and misapprehension. We learned of course the secret signs of Masonic identification for particular use in recognizing unknown fellow members for assistance when in difficulty or danger.

We who were preparing to become Masons found that the Old World symbolism and ritual knowledge united us in a bond of mutual purpose and friendship. These feelings intensified as the days of preparation continued. In the final induction ceremony, in an atmosphere highly charged with the drama and mysticism, the ritual unfolded through ancient signs and symbols, and we jointly committed ourselves to secret trusts and obligations, each to create a new edifice of his own life. Then we chose the name: Light of the

Eastern Star Lodge of Masonic Orders, at Cruzeiro do Sul, Acre Territory, Brazil.

When it was all over I started the long trip up the Rio Moa and overland again to the Rio Tapiche and home at Tamashi Manchari. I had been gone six weeks or so. Soon my induction into the Masonic Order dimmed into memory, to remain only that for many years, but it was of crucial importance to me in a later episode of my life.

Back home Nieves and I started talking more seriously now about leaving the Rio Tapiche. By this time I had children, two daughters to think of and provide for, as well as my wife and myself. Actually it was among my own family and my Indian workers that I began using the medical knowledge I had acquired from living with the Huni Kui. I had prepared herbal baths and extracts for Nieves to drink before and after the birth of our children, there in the forest. And she had no complications from childbirth. But, about the time I returned from Cruzeiro do Sul, the younger of my daughters became ill. She was just learning to talk and so I could not ask her about how she felt to help me determine the source of her trouble, but one day Nieves asked me, "Why do you suppose the ants are attracted to the urinal our daughter uses at night?"

This question triggered a chain of thought that went back to the time I had spent with the Huni Kui as their captive medicine man. I remembered they were very careful not to foul their village with human wastes. Each person had a place in the jungle which he used. Old Chief Xumu, who taught me what I know about jungle medicine, warned his Indians to come and tell him if ants swarmed to a place where one of them urinated. And I also remembered what treatment he gave them when this happened. So I prepared an extract for my daughter to drink from the bark of a special small woody plant, called *ihuashtec*[10] by the Huni Kui, that grows among the bare rocks of the fast-flowing small creeks in the forest. In a few days she was much better and soon all trace of her trouble left.

This same treatment I have used many times since then to relieve serious cases of diabetes, cases that professional doctors have failed to help. One of these patients still takes the remedy I provide from time to time so that his trouble will not return. And new cases are referred to me by patients who have recovered.

Eventually we decided that we would have to leave the headwaters of the Tapiche and locate nearer the main river, the Rio Ucayali. After arranging for our Witoto, Santa Rosa, and Cocama Indians to stay on with Juan Hidalgo, we loaded everything in our biggest canoe and left our home in the forest at Tamashi Manchari. We stopped at the Borda trading post, Callao, to settle our accounts, and then went on to Requena at the mouth of the Tapiche where it flows into the Rio Ucayali.

At Requena one of the first persons I encountered was Padre Agustín Lopez, founder of the Catholic Mission and Convent School for Girls.[11] He reminded me that I had taken my wife from his school without permission or sanction. Now he advised me that the least I could do was get married by the church to protect the future welfare of my wife and children. I agreed wholeheartedly and promptly made arrangements for the ceremony. This official and formal recognition of our marriage added a new dimension to our already close relationship, and the ceremony of course made Nieves and her mother happy. The two girls were baptized, and we also arranged for a memorial mass to be celebrated for Nieves' father, whose disappearance into the forest of the upper Rio Juruá I had helped to explain.

Here at Requena I met Juan Copete, a friend of my Mother's family in Moyobamba. He told me about a place up the Ucayali where there was high ground that did not flood even during high water. It was called Águano Isla, Mahogany Island. Juan said that he intended to leave his camp there on the island to return to Juanjui in the mountains near Moyobamba, and that I could have his squatter's rights to the place. So I left my family with Nieves' mother in Requena and started my hunt for a new home by going up the main river to Águano Isla. This move really brought to an end my life in the forest. Afterward my visits lasted at most only a few months.

7

Life at Águano Isla

FROM REQUENA I WENT UP THE RIO UCAYALI BY LAUNCH TO ÁGUANO Isla with Juan Copete. There he and Abelardo Torres had a camp and the beginnings of a farm, but they didn't like this big flat river country that flooded every year when high water came. They were both from the mountain country around Moyobamba and said they were going back there. But they told me—and it turned out to be true—that Águano Isla was a high *restinga,*[1] a ridge, that did not flood even in years of highest water. And there was lots of game because the animals and birds gathered there when the rest of the country flooded.

I liked the place and decided to take over the camp from the two men. They took me to Juan Arirama, a Cocama Indian living on the upper end of the island. I asked him to make a temporary house where we could stay while I looked the island over for the best home site. He agreed to put up the house as I asked, and I returned to Requena for my family. I remembered later that he had said something to me about tigers or jaguars—that you couldn't keep domestic animals or fowl on the island because the jaguars would eat them—but I gave it little thought.

Soon we were back at Águano Isla with all our worldly belongings, Nieves and I and our two young daughters. The house that Arirama had built was no palace, with its palm roof held up by poles cut from the forest and only an earthen floor, but we were all glad to be in a house of our own again.

I brought chickens and pigs from Requena and these began to disappear. It was no difficult task to find out why; the jaguar tracks were plain to be seen where the lost chickens and pig had wandered into the forest nearby. And we could hear the jaguars coughing nearby at night when they came to look the newcomers over.

We couldn't keep our animals penned up because they had to forage for food. Until I planted corn and other grain we would have nothing to feed them. I went to consult with Juan Arirama, but he said it was hopeless to try to kill all the jaguars nearby because more would simply come in from farther away. He said my friend Copete had tried this and it had failed. About then I began to wonder if Copete was my friend or the jaguar's friend when he brought me to this place. Even the children were in danger. Arirama cautioned me to keep them near the house.

One night in my dreams I recalled how the Huni Kui got rid of jaguars that hung around their garden plots in the forest, scaring the women. They gathered sharp thorns and buried them carefully in the jaguar tracks. These animals when they go twice over the same trail step exactly in their former tracks, and thorns buried carefully in their tracks cause such pain that they go away.

But I had an even better plan. In the river there were plenty of stingrays, so I told Arirama and his friends when they caught any stingrays while fishing to save the poisonous spines off the stinging tail for me. As these stingers were brought in I took them out into the forest around our house and very carefully buried one in the center of the left front foot track of each jaguar trail I could find. If you know the jaguar's habits you can find the places where he stops. And when one of these cats starts off again from a stopping place he always puts his left front foot out for the first step.

The prick of the stingray spine is very painful and in the middle of the pad of the jaguar's starting foot, very inconvenient and upsetting besides. The first night after I put the spines out, the bellowing and screaming out there in the forest made your hair stand on end. And every time I got more spines from the fishermen I put them out farther from the house, with the same result each time. Finally the jaguars gave up and soon they abandoned Águano Isla completely and never came back while we were there, even during high water. Stingray spines were too much for them.

Life on Águano Isla left no time for idling. I was a farmer now, not a rubber cutter. Land had to be cleared for crops and pasture, and we had a permanent home to build.

From a nearby swamp forest I located and felled six large *huacapu*[2] treees suitable for the main columns of the house. These would be set in the ground and had to be rot-resistant. Once they were on the ground I chopped off the thin layer of sapwood and left the large trunks to dry while I gathered the other material. This consisted of long *shapaja*[3] palm fronds for the thatched roof, poles for the rafters, supports and tie-rods. Then I also had to split and spread open a number of *pona*[4] palm trunks for the flooring, and gather lengths of *tamishi* vines for tying it all together. There wasn't a nail in the whole house.

I got Juan Arirama and some of his Cocama Indian neighbors to help me with the house, both in getting the materials together and then in putting it up. We procured all the materials in the dark of the moon;[5] I knew if we did the cutting at any other time the products would be riddled by woodborer holes and would deteriorate too soon. After the construction material had dried out or seasoned properly, the actual building was accomplished in a couple of weeks. Then my family and I moved into a comfortable and serviceable new home, the floor five feet off the ground, woven palm walls, and palm-thatched roof—cool and convenient for a tropical climate. It was located near the river at a good place for the water traffic to stop. My next chore was to clear the river bank of forest so the breeze would come in off the river; also we could signal passing launches if we wanted them to stop.

Soon the farm began to prosper. The soil was good and the nearby forest had plenty of game, especially during the high-water times when animals came there to escape the flooding. People wondered how I did so well, but I worked hard and did things at the right time. From my training with the Indians I always knew where wild game could be obtained. I watched and learned where the manatees or water cows fed on floating grass and other water plants, and they provided excellent meat similar to beef. I watched the lakes and connecting channels and soon learned the rhythm and routes of fish migrations with changing water levels. This made net-fishing productive. At low water the river turtles, the *charapas*[6] and the *taracayas,*[7] came out on the sand bars to lay their eggs. Both the eggs and the turtles were good food and could be sold for cash. The *charapas* came out on the beaches only when a rain storm threatened, so that their tracks to where they laid the eggs would be washed away; the *taracayas* were not this clever.

One dry season Juan Arirama, who lived on the beach at the end of our island, came by and said he'd been chased by a *túnche*, a ghost, when he was out catching turtles and gathering eggs at night on the sand bars. Other people made the same complaint, even saying that they had to jump in the river to get away, but I thought little of it.

I had gathered a few *taracayas* and wanted to get enough to take downriver to Requena or perhaps even to Iquitos to market. Isauro de la Torre lived on a beach nearby, called Ceylon, and I went over to see if I could buy some from him to complete my load. Isauro said he had only a few and didn't want to sell them. When I told him where I was going to catch more for myself, he said I'd better be careful and look out for the *túnche*. I laughed and told him that the *túnche*-whistling brought out the turtles!

It was during a period of moonlight, so that night I took my machete and shotgun about 11 o'clock and went down a long forest trail to the other side of my island where there was a broad sandy beach. The drifting clouds partly covered the moon, and lightning played on some big thunderheads in the distance, but only a faint rolling sound of thunder could be heard where I walked on the beach. A good breeze kept me cool.

I worked hard running down some turtles and tying them up with vines. Then I started back up the beach looking for more. When I came to a big pile of driftwood logs and branches, with the wind fluttering wild cane leaves dried and caught in the trash, I heard a grunting and whistling sound coming from the cane growing on the bank nearby. As I turned to see what made it, the shadow of a passing cloud went by. When the moonlight came out again, there on the beach about a hundred yards away stood a giant apparition. It was at least twelve feet tall with its arms outstretched and its white robe flapping in the wind. I heard a distant rumble of thunder and a whistle, then a long 'whoooo-whoooooo' from the monster. The hair stood up on the back of my head and neck. But I held my ground. The *túnche* kind of bowed and stepped out on the beach toward me, whooooooing again and bowing as he came on toward me. Still I held my ground, suspecting a trick, since I did not believe in ghosts.

When the *túnche* hesitated about fifty feet away I raised my shotgun and shouted, "Whatever is inside that thing is going to die with buckshot."

Then I got an answer, "Oh, *compadre*, don't shoot, don't shoot. You'll kill me."

I began to laugh because I recognized the voice, and out of the robes came Isauro de la Torre, dropping on the sand a big cross draped in white cloth made to look like a ghost, a *túnche*. He ran up and embraced me and said again "Don't shoot, don't shoot."

It came out that for a long time he had been scaring people away and stealing the turtles they had gathered on this beach. But now the game was up. He asked me not to denounce him to the authorities, and I did not. But I told my neighbors, including Juan Arirama, that they did not have to fear ghosts any more on the sand bars of Águano Isla, the best turtle-hunting beaches in the neighborhood. Isauro had to move away because the people razzed him so much, especially those that he had scared and robbed of their turtles.

One of our early visitors on Águano Isla was Father Agustín Lopez Pardo, the priest of Requena whom I've already mentioned. He was always traveling up and down the river getting local support for his convent school for girls there in Requena, selecting students, and performing religious functions in the river villages that were without resident priests. Our place was about midpoint on his travels upriver from Requena, and Padre Agustín soon found out that Nieves' house with its ample space and the good cooking made a convenient place to rest up from his arduous river trips. He was always welcome.

Padre Agustín traveled with gear packed in two large cedar-wood chests. When he arrived at our house he would turn these over to Nieves to re-organize the contents. Inside, his robes and clothing would be all thrown together and mixed up with dried salt fish, smoked game, leaking bags of rice and beans, record books, and other impedimentia of river travel. Nieves would wash and mend the clothing and rearrange everything in an orderly way, hoping it would stay that way until he came again. But the chests were always the same when he arrived—a jumbled mess.

We had long discussions, the Padre and I. One day I came in from felling a piece of forest for a new plantation and found that Padre Agustín had just arrived. I was hot and exhausted, my work clothes dripping with the sweat that accompanied any exertion in this hot, humid tropical climate. Before going to the river bank for a bath and change of clothes, I had a cup of coffee with him. "Father Agustín," I asked, "how can I believe in God, when I have to work so hard to make such a miserable living?"

"Ah, my son," he replied, "you completely misunderstand the meaning of God. It is His Presence that makes it possible for you to utilize the fruits of the earth and multiply them for your needs. Give thanks and be grateful."

A wise old man, Padre Agustín—we had many long involved religious discussions. I don't think he realized that I was a Mason, but not much else escaped him. What the relationship is between the Church and the Masonic Orders in other regions I don't know, but in the Latin countries the Church has persistently tried to suppress any threat to its authority. This effort has included the Masons from the time of the founding of the Church in Rome and perhaps even earlier.

While Padre Agustín stayed with us I would take him around to the nearby settlements. One time, I remember, he removed his prayer and record books from his wooden chest and went to a village while I watched the canoe. In the chest were spare vestments. For devilment I donned one of the long black robes and climbed up the river bank where I could see a wide expanse of river. There, standing on an exposed point, I waved and shouted at the passing boats and canoes, calling out "*Misa, misa;* come to mass," and waving my arm for them to come. Most of the people going by recognized me and waved back, laughing. But I was not careful enough in my joke. The Padre saw me as he returned, and he gave me a good lecture on the evils of impersonating a representative of the Church.

During the four years that we lived on the upper Rio Tapiche our first two children were born. When the second child also was a girl I began to worry about having sons and so I decided to go through the ceremony used by the Huni Kui husband who wanted to assure that his next offspring would be male. After the second daughter's birth at Tamishi Manchari I took the placenta off into the forest, dug a hole, and, with proper incantations, jabbed the placenta several times with a spear made out of very hard wood especially for this purpose. Then I broke the spear and buried it with the placenta in the hole. Soon after our arrival at Águano Isla, my first son, Manuel, was born. The next child was also a boy, Jorge. Nieves always took my herbal preparations both before and after the birth of each of our ten children (five girls and five boys), and she had no complications from childbirth. To the children, especially the boys, I gave special herbal baths and other treatments to make them strong and brave. These produced good results. Jorge in fact later became the middle-weight boxing champion of South America, defending his title in Buenos Aires. After that fight Nieves insisted he must stop boxing before he killed someone, and Jorge did stop, to please his mother.

It was during this time when we lived at Águano Isla that I really began to use my healing powers. The people living on the river at that time had little, if any, access to trained doctors. And, in the rough life we all lived, there was plenty of illness. Only those with a strong or superior physique managed to survive. When it became known by word of mouth that I could cure people they came from far and near for help. Most of the cases I cannot even remember anymore.

One case I do remember was the son of a friend, Mariano Cardenas of Puerto Loreto: he had a very bad skin eruption all over his body, and everyone around thought he had leprosy. At his father's request I examined the boy carefully and started treatment with various purges and baths. In three months he recovered completely. Apparently he had a form of pellagra resulting from a bad diet and complicated by taking the wrong medicine. He was in very bad condition with terrible skin sores when I undertook treatment.

He certainly could not have lived much longer, and his family was very grateful to me for his recovery.

After we were well established at Águano Isla and had been there two or three years the river currents changed. Especially during the annual high water stage of the river, the bank where our house was located began to erode away. With a stream the size of the Ucayali there is nothing you can do to fight or hold the river. The laws of hydraulics rule. Even the best engineers from North America and Holland have not stopped the river-front buildings of Iquitos from tumbling into the river as the bank of my home town now erodes away.

It got so bad there at Águano Isla that during one time of high water we had to move everything hurriedly out of our house—quickly building a temporary shelter, and then a whole new house. Great chunks of the forest caved into the river, each with a roar like that of a big wind, and huge trees just disappeared into tremendous irresistible river currents. I feared our house would go this way some night, taking us all into the raging water too.

I was in the middle of building a new house and moving our things when an Indian paddled his canoe into our landing from somewhere upriver. His woman was with him and she sat in the canoe while the man climbed up the steps and came to where I was working on the new house. I could tell that he was in trouble from the way he approached. He came right to the point, saying "My wife gave birth several days ago and we cannot stop the flow of blood. They told us upriver that you could help her."

"Look," I said, "my house is falling into the river and my family is out in the rain. I am in the middle of building a new house and moving. More rain is coming. How can I stop now?"

"But my wife is dying—bleeding to death, and they told me upriver you could save her," came the Indian's subdued reply.

I could never turn suffering people away when I had it in my power to help, so I said, "Well, we can try. Where is she?" and the Indian pointed to the canoe below the river bank.

"Bring her up," I told him. "Make a roof here with these palm leaves and poles. We have no house to offer, as you can see. I will have to go into the forest to collect the necessary plants. But bring your wife up first, so I can see her."

The Indian went to the canoe, gathered the limp bundle that was his wife into his arms and brought her up the bank. She was too weak to walk. Nieves put some bedding on the ground for her to lie on, and I asked, "Where is the baby?"

"Upriver with friends. It is healthy but she could not feed it."

The pale, drawn girl just lay on the ground with her eyes closed, saying nothing, not even moving. She hardly seemed to breathe as I looked down at her.

Rain was coming; I could see the clouds building up and feel a change in the air that meant a storm. So I picked up my machete, told the man again to fix a shelter with the palm fronds, and walked off in the direction of the forest. I needed a vine, bark of a certain tree, and leaves of a shrub to stop the uterine bleeding. Within an hour I was back and had them boiling over a fire. This process you cannot hurry if you expect results. But as soon as it was ready I gave a large bottle of warm, dark liquid to the Indian and said within hearing of the girl, "Have her drink a small cupful about every hour until it is all gone. This will help her."

Then we all had to scramble to get our things under cover of the partial roof of our new house because a deluge of rain had started. Later in the evening Nieves and I took some food over to the visitors' lean-to. The young woman opened her eyes and barely managed a small smile. She looked somewhat better already.

Thunder, wind, and rain lasted the whole night, but when Nieves took a pot of coffee to them in the morning the woman was sitting up, looking much better. She held out the empty bottle for us to see.

That afternoon she told Nieves, "In the night during the wind and rain I had a dream or vision. I saw a large black serpent leave my body and after it was gone I felt the blood stop flowing out. Don Manuel has taken the evil spirit out of my body and saved my life."

The next day the Indian couple left and went back upriver. And with them another story began the rounds of how I had saved a life with plants from the forest.

About this time a young man from across the river, Purificacíon Ramírez, started helping me on the farm. My stories of life with the Indians fascinated him and he asked me to teach him how to prepare and use my jungle remedies. Well, it's not so simple a matter as just showing someone how to gather bark or leaves from the forest and put them to boil. But somehow there seemed implicit in my training with old Chief Xumu a mandate to pass the learning on to someone who could continue its application after my time. And with this obligation implanted in my mind by the old chief, I undertook the indoctrination and training of an apprentice.

I tried to set up a training regime for young Ramírez, similar to the one I had gone through, but it proved impossible. I could not control his diet nor his activites as the chief had restricted mine off there in that isolated Indian village deep in the forest. It seemed that about the time we would reach some crucial point in the training Ramírez would always make an excuse to go off somewhere. These breaks in the continuity of training demonstrated a certain lack of mental discipline. That is perhaps the reason my disciple never quite seemed to gain control of the visions. He could not direct their flow to discover the source of the illness of a patient nor determine the plant preparations appropriate for the cure. He seemed to think all he had to do was imitate me, but that of course was not enough. After a couple of years we gave it up and he left.

Somehow Ramírez' cures were ineffective even when he prepared his medicine from the same plants that I had taught him to use. He never seemed to be able properly to integrate the needs of his patients with the properties of the plants he used nor could he organize an adequate system of treatment. His efforts proved superficial; he could not grasp the fundamentals. No doubt a large part of the cause for failure came from my lack of control over the circumstances surrounding our efforts. At this time José Ríos-Ríos came to live with us from Moyobamba, as an orphaned youngster. He always hung around when I was trying to train Ramírez, and learned just enough to get himself into trouble later with the Murato Indians on the Rio Corrientes. We heard, remember, during our Rio Tigre survey how the Muratos killed him for practicing witchcraft on them—the result of misapplied knowledge.

The river, during this time, inexorably kept changing its course and eating into our island. On one of his trips Padre Agustín stopped for several days to rest with us and I showed him the problem we were having with the river. It was obvious from the way the current was cutting into the bank that we would have to move our house again soon.

Padre Agustín said to me, "I have been traveling and observing the river for more than twenty-five years. Its changes are unpredictable and beyond control. You have a family now that will need an education and some security. On this part of the river there is no security, no way to educate your sons and daughters. I think you should take your family to Iquitos."

We did not move in a hurry. But I observed the river and made other plans. On a trip to Iquitos to sell some produce from my fields I sought out a boyhood friend with whom I had gone to school. Ferucho Gabriel Cortez owned the cockfighting ring in Iquitos and he invited me to go into partnership with him. He had many other commercial and legal affairs to take care of and said he did not have time to look after the ring and the fighting cocks properly. So, in a few months, while the river continued to cave in the bank in front of my house on Águano Isla, I sold off all my livestock and my plantation and when this was done we moved to Iquitos.

Since we left, the river has completely eroded away Águano Isla. Nothing remains to show where we lived all those years. The habitation nearest to it is another riverbank village now called La Perlita. Padre Agustín gave me good advice when he suggested that we move to Iquitos, just as he did when he recommended that I get married.

8

Fighting Cocks

IN LATE 1929, WHEN I WAS FORTY-ONE YEARS OLD, I MOVED MY FAMILY TO Iquitos. There I bought a half interest in the Cortez cockfighting gallery and immersed myself in the intricate business of building up its fame. Gabriel, after a few months, decided he wanted to liquidate his interests in Iquitos and move to Lima; thus I bought out his half interest and rebuilt the Córdova *Coliseo de Gallos* on my own property on Calle Napo where I could maintain closer control.

As sole owner of the cockfighting establishment I made my money in a number of ways. It came from the small entrance fees charged the spectators, from the fees charged for entering cocks in fights, from a twenty percent house charge on all wagers made on fights, and from the sale of refreshments. I turned the refreshment stand over to my boys Manuel and Jorge. They sold fresh fruit drinks, sandwiches, sweets, and othe snacks through a supply arrangement made with their mother. This kept them in spending money and more. But the over-all success of a cockfight pit is tied in with owning a top-flight string of fighting cocks which can be matched against all comers put up to fight by other *aficionados*, and the real money comes from the betting, for I could also make wagers on these in-house fighting cocks. There are many opportunities to place bets both before and during a fight. Odds against one bird and for another fluctuate constantly during a fight. This is all communicated, along with bets going back and forth around the pit and in the stands, by means of hand and finger signals flashing at lightning speed. These make up a special language of the game. At the climax of a fight between two well-matched roosters there is a welling up of frenzied, hoarse shouting as each spectator urges on his favorite combatant.

By purchase, trade, selection, and elimination I soon had a crack string of cocks that drew attention of *aficionados* in several countries. I developed connections for exchange of birds with other ring owners in Peru, especially in Chiclayo and Lima, and outside the country in Guayaquil, Ecuador, and in the Colombian cities of Leticia and Bogota. But one of the most advantageous contacts I had was with a Brazilian friend, Joaquin de Melo Nieto. He held the position of postal clerk on one of the Brazilian ships that came to Iquitos from European and South American ports. Melo brought me choice fighting cocks and breeding pullets from Manaus, Belem, Rio de Janeiro, and from Buenos Aires. Occasionaly his ship would go to Hamburg, Germany, and from there Melo obtained breeding stock from the best blood lines of Malayan and Japanese fighting cocks which he brought to me.

Of course I could not give my friend money for the friendship he showed in bringing me these choice fighting cocks and pullets from around the world. This was Melo's way of expressing *cariño*, his high regard for me, always above the level of money. But I naturally wanted to express my appreciation, so I obtained from Moyobamba and Rioja the very choicest, finely woven straw hats. The Indians in those two towns of San Martín Province weave a *sombrero* finer than even the best of the world-famous Panama hats (that are actually woven in Ecuador). The Moyobamba hat is a true work of the weaver's art, and I am sure that *amigo* Melo disposed of my friendly offerings to his own advantage one way or another in compensation for feeding chickens on his long voyages across the sea.

In Iquitos, cockfights were held only one day a week, on Sunday. And as rivalry built up around town to try to overcome the superiority of my fighting cocks, the gallery filled up every Sunday.

One of the best fighters I ever had Melo brought me from Hamburg when the rooster was about fourteen months old and before he had ever been matched in the pit for a fight. This young *gallo* would dance about on his toes, bob his head around, ruffle his feathers and crow, giving all the signs and signals of real fighting promise. I trained him well on the running table to strengthen his legs, tossed him back and forth from one hand to the other catching him by the breast to build up his wing muscles. And with chamois leather pads bound on his heel spurs I tested him in sparring matches with some of my other top fighters. His first fight in the pit was so explosive the spectators shouted out "Dynamite! Dynamite!" and from then on Dynamite was his name.

With my training, Dynamite became what we called a "high flyer." He could rise eight to ten feet in the air from a standing start. No opponent ever rose above him, but if an adversary came up anywhere near, Dynamite flailed him with wings and cut him by churning, lethal spurs. Dynamite's matches seldom went beyond three or four passes; by then he had dominated and dispatched his opponent.

For fighting power and stamina in the pit I fed my cocks on the Saturday before a match only a cupful of chopped liver steeped in vinegar. Other days they had cracked grain, green forage, and scratch of ground shells and sifted charcoal. This diet kept them in top form.

Dynamite brought fame to my cockfighting gallery. His conquests were talked about among *aficionados* all over Peru and even farther away. Everything put in the ring with Dynamite was dispatched in such spectacular fashion that soon no one would put up an opponent against him. After breeding him to several pullets to preserve the fighting bloodline, I sold him to a friend in the cockfighting center of Chiclayo on the Peruvian coast. Later he was sold again, when no more opponents could be found in Chiclayo, and taken to Ecuador. Then I lost track of him.

Other famous fighters starting their careers in my string went by the names of Capitan Sangre, Trak-Trak, and Volador. These all went on to fight in other centers and brought attention to their place of origin: Córdova's *Coliseo de Gallos* at Iquitos. In connection with any cockfighting gallery there is continually a ferment of intrigue and rivalry—my place was no exception. Someone was always, by fair scheme or foul, trying to get ahead of you by winning, and often tempers flared. To keep order and avoid outright fist fights between participants, bettors, and spectators, I always had at least one uniformed policeman in attendance.

The breeding, training, and conditioning of game fowl is no occupation for a lazy man and I had all the problems of running the fighting gallery as well. This took lots of time and plenty of hard work. But more than cockfighting claimed my attention in Iquitos. Word of my ability to heal the sick and suffering followed me from upriver by word of mouth and grew with each new healing success.

A friend of ours, Ana Delgado de Menada, had an Indian servant girl who the doctors warned should be dismissed. They said she had tuberculosis and there was danger of infecting the household. But Doña Ana knew the girl would have no place else to go since she had never worked for anyone else, and the Indian village from which she had been stolen probably no longer existed. She could not return there.

Doña Ana came to me and asked me to look at the girl, which I did. When she coughed and spit blood I asked her to spit in a pan of water. The blood spread out on top of the water but did not sink in globules as happens in the case of tuberculosis. After this I sat down and questioned her very carefully about how her trouble started. The girl was very weak now, had a fever, and had lost confidence in everyone, especially doctors.

Finally with patience I drew her out and found that several months before she had stepped on a piece of rusty barbed wire. The cut had healed but a week or two later a sore knot had appeared behind her knee, then one in the groin, and finally one in her armpit. The infection finally settled in her lungs, causing her to spit blood. This prompted the doctors to guess she had tuberculosis, but treatment for that disease certainly was no help to her.

I started her soaking the pierced foot in hot salt water and gave her drinking water in which *retama*[1] flowers had been boiled. After several hours of bathing, the foot softened up. In a day or two the old cut opened and a large quantity of pus drained out. I had her continue bathing it off and on for several days until the draining stopped and the infection was cleared up. Then I gave her an herb tonic which brought back her appetite and helped her recover strength. In a few weeks she was fully recovered. Of course Doña Ana was greatly relieved and very grateful to me for having the girl well again.

Doña Ana was a friend of the local Superior Court Justice and when his daughter, married to a young pilot in the Peruvian Air Force, was dying, she urged the judge to consult with me. They called me to the Justice's home here in Iquitos and he asked me to examine his daughter. She had been under the constant care of three doctors for over a year, he told me. Now they informed him they could do nothing more for her and that she was dying.

"I will have to see her alone, or at least without the presence of persons who believe what the doctors have told you," I said to the judge.

"Whatever you say," he replied, "you are our only hope now."

He took me to the bedroom and I stayed for a while talking quietly but confidently with the girl. Her great luminous eyes told me she had plenty of vitality left, but it is true that without help she was close to death. Indeed, many of my patients have come to me only after the doctors have given up. Now I asked the girl only a few questions about how her condition had begun—what had caused her to see a doctor at first. When I rose to go and told her I would be back the following day with something to help her recover, she smiled and I knew then that she could be cured.

When I got home I told Nieves to fix me only roast chicken breast for supper. She looked at me and said, "Oh, you want me to sit with you tonight?" She knew the signs very well.

"Yes, and send the young ones to spend the night with their sister. I want absolute quiet in the house tonight."

Then I went to my workroom and started boiling slowly, in a special pot used for nothing else, a section of the *ayahuasca* vine with leaves of *chacruna*, using the proper chants. By midnight the liquid would be settled and cool. The street noise and other disturbances here on Jiron Huallaga where I live now are too great, even late at night, for a good *ayahuasca* vision session. But no matter, I no longer require the stimulation of the vision vine extract to determine my cures. When the case of the judge's daughter came to my attention, back before the war, we lived on Calle Napo. Our house had an upstairs room at the back with windows overlooking a grassy playing field which merged on the far side into the forest. There in that room you could completely isolate yourself from any kind of neighborhood disturbance. And a night breeze from the forest kept the room pleasantly cool.

At about 11 p.m., when the neighborhood had quieted down, we went to that upper back room in the Calle Napo house. Our only light was a small candle with the flame shaded from our eyes. Nieves sat down in her cane rocker, as she had done numerous times before, and prepared for an all-night vigil.

From a small clay jar made especially for me many years ago by a Capanahua Indian woman, I poured a cupful of greenish-brown liquid, taking great care to disturb the fluid as little as possible. Calmly then I drank down in one draft this slightly bitter extract of the vision vine, *ayahuasca*, which I had prepared with my own hands. Lying back, relaxed, in my hammock strung between iron rings set in the wall, I chanted softly to myself, thus focusing my attention on the patient I had been called in to see that same morning. In this way I awaited and guided the sequence of events I had learned to control.

Amigo, I have described to you before what happens—a soft ringing in the ears, sometimes a slight muscular shock, and then color visions progressing into a shimmering golden aura. Using the technique ingrained into me by my training with the old Indian chief, Xumu—with songs and chants that I only half remembered afterwards—I directed the course of my visions to my young patient. In the heightened state of perception brought on by my trance, every function of her body was apparent to me. In infinite detail her internal organs appeared on the screen of my vision. As the liver came to my sight, it was obvious from its black color that it had ceased to function and I knew it was no longer serving to purify the blood. As this became clear to me I turned my attention to the remedy, and the appropriate plants appeared in my vision—flowers from the *retama* tree and roots from the *retamilla*[2] shrub. As the visions faded off into more general dreams I knew it was possible for her to recover.

It was the next morning at breakfast that Nieves startled me. "As you lay there last night mumbling and chanting to yourself," she said, "I dozed for a bit in my rocking chair, and I saw some of your visions. That poor girl—she looked like the judge's daughter—and her liver was so swollen and black! And then I saw some kind of flowers—what were they? I hope you can make that poor girl well again."

Now you will wonder, as I do. How could Nieves, sitting there with me at night, have captured and described so well the next morning the content of my *ayahuasca* visions? I had not told her anything about the case, not even what house I had visited the day before. For a moment I could only look at her in astonishment. "It's true!" she said, "I saw your visions."

Well at that point I did not have time to speculate on the marvels of *ayahuasca* which had surprised me many times before with its revelations, although I have pondered this transmission of my visions since. Now I had a dying patient to treat. I had promised help on this very day, and the plant extracts which were needed would take time to prepare properly.

First I had to detoxify the girl from all the months of improper medication she had received. I did this with a very mild extract from the roots of the *retamilla* shrub. When I took this to my patient I told her mother to give her daughter a drink of this whenever she was thirsty, saying with strong assurance that it would help her. And true enough, in only a few days the judge's daughter was showing marked improvement, and I told them to begin to give her light nourishment in the form of soup. Then I prepared an extract by boiling dried *retama* flowers. Taking this liquid caused further improvement. Within a month the young woman was taking *chuchuhuasha*[3] tree-bark extract to stimulate her appetite and speed her recovery. In another month complete recovery was in sight. A miracle, everyone said, but actually there was no medical reason for her condition. Proper diagnosis and treatment of early symptoms would have avoided the deathbed conditions I had to deal with.

The judge was extremely grateful to me for his daughter's recovery from what had appeared to be her deathbed to a condition of radiant health. Later he was transferred to the Court of Moyobamba. When I had some serious trouble with the local authorities, I heard that he had offered to return to Iquitos to defend me in court. But the problem was solved another way.

My success both in healing patients whom the local medical men failed to help and my financial gain from the cockfighting ring were resented by some people. My income from healing people amounted to little because I charged only a token of the treatment's value. But there was a flaw in my position which made me vulnerable to exploitation and persecution by unscrupulous individuals. I had no license to practice medicine.

The large affairs of men often turn on small events. One day a fiscal inspector came by and asked to see my license to operate the cockfighting ring. I showed him the license Ferucho had transferred to me when I bought out his half of the partnership. As the inspector looked at it he said, "But you have moved it to a new location. This is for the old ring." I replied that as it was the same business, the license remained valid. He returned the paper to me and departed without further comment.

I asked a few discreet questions at the *Alcaldia* (Municipal Offices), but got only evasive answers and was about to forget the whole affair. But then during a night of disturbed sleep I had a repeat of a wild dream that had first come to me years ago when I lived off there in the forest with the Indians.

In this dream I found myself wandering alone in a forest of tremendous trees. Rough misshapen boulders, twisting vines, and other hideous defilements of the jungle lurked everywhere and the ground was an uneven slippery morass. The sound of a hauntingly strange birdcall held my attention. In the silence as the call faded I heard the twang of a plucked bow string. A tremendous feathered arrow came hurtling through the air directly at me. I stood transfixed, unable to move. The missile struck me down and a replusive grimacing savage stepped out from behind a tree. His immense body, painted a vivid red, seemed to pulsate with strength and energy as he stepped to where I lay on the ground. Deliberately he put a naked foot on my chest as my lifeblood ebbed out onto the ground—here, as before, the dream ended. And as before, the nightmarish vision during my sleep left me depressed and uneasy for some days.

And on one fateful day in my life, not long after my nightmare, a messenger from the local court came to my house and said the *vocál*, the speaker of the Superior Court, one Cedron, wanted to see me. Then I knew there was trouble brewing, but I ignored the summons. It just happens that Cedron, before coming to Iquitos, had been speaker of the Court in Moyobamba and had been forced to leave there for abuse of his position. I had friends and relatives in Moyobamba because that is where my mother came from, so I had some inkling of what to expect of the situation that was developing.

In an hour or two the messenger came again and repeated the summons. And again I ignored the message, but I began to seethe with anger. Soon this fellow was back for the third time, saying if I did not come the police would be sent to bring me. I knew this was an idle threat, but I decided I would have to go confront the situation. When I arrived at the office of the court, Cedron immediately started the vilification. "Who do you think you are, to ignore my summons?" he shouted.

"You have no authority to summon me," I replied.

"You will find out who has authority around here. You are exploiting the people with your fraudulent practice of medicine. You've got no license to practice medicine. You're nothing but a fraud! And I'll see that you're prosecuted for it."

This accusation of fraud struck me like the branding of a red hot iron, and I reacted spontaneously and violently! We were facing one another and as he finished speaking I drew back and gave him the full impact of a clenched fist on the side of his jaw. I was not exactly a weakling and he went sprawling to the floor, screaming obscenities at me, and I shouted back, "If you want more, just call me here again!" Then I strode out of there before he could get up. He needed help.

I went right back home, becoming more agitated every step of the way. When I arrived home and Nieves saw me, a look of horror crossed her face. She had never before seen my Indian-trained fighting instincts aroused.

Word of this incident spread like wildfire through Iquitos. A friend and patient, also a *vocál* or court speaker, sent word that I should go into hiding immediately until the situation quieted down. He said that I should by all means avoid arrest, that Cedron would undoubtedly send the police to arrest me.

When this message came I gathered up some things in a small valise and under cover of darkness went to a friend's farmhouse several miles outside Iquitos at Morona Cocha. I told only my oldest son where I was going and warned him to be careful not to be followed if he brought me any messages.

In a day or two a note came from my friend the Comandante of the Civil Guard, saying that the situation was so complicated by the fact that I had struck the Court speaker that he recommended I go to Brazil for a few months until my friends could get things under control again.

In another few days I got the message that a Brazilian launch was in port and that arrangements were being made for it to take me to Brazil. Late one night I went to say good-bye to my family, then boarded the launch at the dock as the gangplank was being pulled up.

9

Exile and Return

AS THE LAUNCH PULLED AWAY AND THE LIGHTS OF IQUITOS FADED INTO the night my feelings were mixed—a certain sense of relief knowing that I would not disgrace my family by going to jail, but outraged at having to run away from an unjust accusation that my impulsive reaction had enlarged into a *causa célebre*. I could see problems looming in the future. First of all I had no documents for legally entering Brazil, and second, how would I support myself and send something back to maintain my family? Fortunately Manuel my eldest son was mature and intelligent enough to run the cockfighting ring. He had been helping me, and I had given him advice and instructions before leaving. Also, my friends and allies in Iquitos would help protect him from predators.

At the first meal on board where the passengers sat down at the table I looked at the Captain and gave him the secret handsign of the Masonic Lodge. He responded and immediately I knew that I had a trusted ally. After the meal he took me to his cabin and asked what he could do for me.

I told him the story of my departure and he replied, "Be at ease. You are among friends now, or will be as soon as we cross the border into Brazil. As a fellow Mason you have no problems that we cannot take care of." He insisted that I use his cabin during the trip and took his things to other quarters.

At the port of exit from Peru, a place called Ramon Castillo, the Captain went personally to the authorities and arranged for my exit without complications and did the same to take care of my entry into Brazil at Benjamin Constant.

When we arrived at Manaus, the Captain of the Port came out

for customs inspection. As soon as he saw my opened bag with the Masonic insignia on the inside of the cover he asked me to close the bag and wait until he had finished with the other passengers. He came to the Captain's cabin when through with his inspection and we exchanged the Masonic handshake as the Captain introduced him. "Limirio Araújo da Sosa, Captain of the Port of Manaus, at your service," he said. The launch captain briefly explained the circumstances of my departure from Iquitos and Captain Araújo said to me, "Consider Manaus your home. I personally will arrange your Brazilian identification papers. The Peruvian consul here is a friend of mine and he will take care of your Peruvian documents any time I ask him. And for the time being, you will be my guest, living at my residence."

We went ashore to Manaus, a place that I had not seen since my youth when I passed this way on my way home after escaping from the Indians on the upper Rio Purus. Great changes were evident in the city, and I certainly had the feeling that for myself the best had been made of a difficult situation.

Soon I was introduced to other fellow Masons, and of course they asked where I had become a Mason. When I told them, they sent a telegram to my friend Alfredo Mancio Lima in Cruzeiro do Sul. He replied of course that I was a founding member of the Eastern Star Lodge there in Cruzeiro do Sul, and from that day on any problems that might have developed for me in Manaus were all solved or taken care of for as long as I might stay.

When the Captain of the Port, Araújo, found out that I was interested in medicine he invited the doctors who belonged to the Manaus Masonic Lodge to his home to discuss and exchange medical experiences with me. These men expressed surprise at my grasp of medical minutiae without formal training in the profession. This was my first close association with men trained in medicine and I took advantage of the free exchange of ideas and information to improve and formalize my vocabulary of human anatomy, bodily functions, and human disease. These men were amazed at my descriptions of internal organs and their functions, things they knew from courses in anatomy and dissection in medical school. Their surprise turned to admiration and respect when I accompanied some of them on their rounds to the wards of a local hospital. In the tubercular ward I pointed out several patients who were being treated erroneously for tuberculosis, when that was not the cause of their illness. Later, after further diagnosis proved that I was correct in my judgment and the treatment I suggested proved effective, my position in medical circles in Manaus became firmly established.

I had long discussions on the medicinal properties of the Amazonian flora with doctors Limirio da Costa and Mitrides de Lima Correa who were both Masons. Even though these doctors were trained in European medical schools, the names of which I forget, the native flora made up an important source of their *materia medica*. The more we discussed the diagnosis of illness and curing with substances derived from the Amazonian flora, the more I realized that in many ways my knowledge was superior to theirs. During our conversations, among many other things, I explained how to use effectively an extract from the bark of a tree called in Peru *tahuari negro*[1]—this was *pau d'arco*[2] in Brazil—for the treatment of abdominal tumors. Naturally my friends wanted to test the preparation themselves. I was unsuccessful in finding the right variety of the tree locally but told my doctor friends that it grew in the forests of the highland country of the upper Rios Purus and Juruá where I had lived with my Indians. After that I forgot all about the incident. But my colleagues did not forget, because later after I had returned to Peru, through the intermediary of the company I worked for, they requested a large sample of the Peruvian *tahuari* bark for testing in Manaus.

Before long I had a small practice of healing of my own there without any persecution from the local authorities. No one in Manaus objected to my making sick people well. But the Masonic Lodge was my main focal point of interest and orientation during my exile. The members encouraged me to advance beyond the beginning grade of my initiation in Cruzeiro do Sul. With their guidance and support I began a program of diligent study to master the ritual and wisdom required to progress through the ancient orders of the builders in stone. This work was of great importance to me in adjusting to my exile. The philosophical teaching of Freemasonry became an important influence on the further development of my healing practice. The symbolism of Masonry as I came to understand and accept it represented both a quest for knowledge and a program of self-improvement and inner transformation. By study and the counselling of more advanced fellow members, I realized that it was possible to transform the edifice of my life and to integrate my jungle training with the esoteric wisdom of my ancestors. I was taught to lay aside the past and take up a new body of intention, desire, and purpose. In myself I was reborn. Symbolically, the keystone of highest esteem must be lost, sought, and found again. No matter how far I had already come, I had to return there by new means. In work and service, not ritual alone, are the realization of Masonry, and also its true attainments.

As I immersed myself in these teachings the use of my knowledge of healing gradually emerged as a personal commitment and the mission of my life. Increasing awareness of the uncommon nature of my medical lore came from association with these men in Manaus, men formally trained in the profession of medicine. And with this realization of the worth of my healing gift, there surfaced again that sense of obligation planted in my mind by my original teacher, old Chief Xumu. Toward the end of his life Xumu made clear his feeling that he could not depart this world of the living until he had adequately trained a successor. Because of his influence on my life it was natural that I should have something of the same feeling.

Many Peruvians traveled back and forth between Manaus and Iquitos. Soon, through them, I communicated with my family in Iquitos. I learned that Cedron had died not long after our violent confrontation, and the doctor who collaborated with him in my denunciation had been forced to leave Iquitos when the connection became known. Luis Felipe Morey, my patient and friend, also a Speaker of the Superior Court, told me later he had warned Cedron that it had been a serious mistake on his part to accuse me of doing anything wrong. As the affair turned out he was right—Cedron dead and his collaborator forced to move away.

In Manaus I met Douglas Allen, president of the American company, Astoria, which had operations to extract commercial products from the Amazon forest in both Peru and Brazil. It was through Astoria and other friends in Peru that the way was cleared for my return home. Mr. Allen showed great interest in my knowledge of the medicinal plants of the forest and offered me a position with Compania Astoria Peruana—to undertake a collection of plants for the company. This collection, he said, was to serve as a basis for developing commercial medical products. I looked forward to this work with satisfaction, and hoped it would lead to understanding and perpetuation of the knowledge I had accumulated at such risk from a source which probably no longer exists.

My Brazilian friends and mentors, when they found I planned to return home, used every persuasive device they could think of to convince me that I should remain. But as with my unplanned stay with the Indians, when I became convinced that it was time to go home, nothing could deter me for long. My gratitude for the treatment and acceptance I received from people in high positions in Manaus is beyond expression. But when the time came, I had to go. They all realized this and released me with good will and understanding.

With a feeling of great anticipation and joy I returned home to my family. Though I had been gone only two years it seemed more like half a century and it was a great day in Casa Córdova when I returned from Manaus. I had to get acquainted with the younger children all over again, they had grown and changed so much. Nieves and the two older boys had done a good job of managing affairs while I had been away and this was a great source of pride.

Before leaving Manaus I had been told by Mr. Allen that my first job when I went to work for the Astoria Company in Iquitos would be to assist the company in the investigation of medicinal plants of the Amazon forest. I knew this would require long field trips into the forest and that I could not manage the cockfighting ring as before. My sons, after all, had to be released now to their own affairs. Therefore, I decided to sell the Córdova *Coliseo de Gallos*. José O'Neil, general manager of Astoria, questioned my wisdom in selling it, but I told him an employee with too many bosses was no good to anyone and he accepted the truth of that. With the money from the sale I bought this house on Jiron Huallaga, where I have lived ever since.

Before I began my botanical explorations, which the Company hoped would lead to commercial use of some of the medicinal plants of the Amazon, I was given detailed instruction on how to prepare botanical specimens in the Iquitos office. They directed me to make a complete collection of all medicinal plants which I considered to have commercial prospects, each specimen to include leaves, flowers, fruit, bark, and other important parts of the plant. This material, they said, would then be scientifically identified, analyzed, and the results published for the benefit of medical science—in Peru and elsewhere.

Astoria had begun in Peru as a sawmilling and mahogany lumber exporting enterprise. This activity had always been the main source of income, so there was considerable snickering and joking around the office about the work of *el botanico*, the botanist. Especially Muñoz, in charge of the office—he was always trying to divert me to running insignificant errands for him when I was busy in the back room preparing the botanical specimens for shipment to New York.

Two long years it took to collect the plants from the forest and prepare the material for shipment according to requirements. It was not easy to find the plants I wanted at times when they were in flower or fruit. Naturally I could not go back to collect plants where I had acquired most of my knowledge about them—there in the land of the Huni Kui at the headwaters of the Rio Purus and Rio de las Piedras. So I went to the next best area that I knew, the upland forest of the Rio Tapiche headwaters.

The company obtained for my use a roomy metal boat and equipped it with an outboard motor. The boat was named, appropriately enough, *El Botanico*, the letters painted on the bow nameplate. In this vessel I went up the Tapiche; in a way it was like returning home. As I have said before, the forests of the upper Tapiche River are one of my favorite areas. But I found the river nearly abandoned, except for a few seasonal camps used by mahogany log producers.

The Capanahua Indians had all moved west to the headwaters of the Rio Buncuya. My Indians—the Witoto Seguas, Santa Rosa Mañanitas, and the Cocama Iraricas—had returned to their native areas of the Putumayo and Napo Rivers, at least according to the few people who were still living on the river from the rubber boom days.

It required several extended trips to the Rio Tapiche headwaters to complete my medicinal plant collection. When I came back from each field trip the plants I had collected were carefully dried and packaged for shipment to New York with a report[3] on their medical properties compiled from my knowledge and experience with patients. Two large wooden boxes with several hundred plant specimens in them were shipped to New York. This completed my first project with the company.

Going back to the Rio Tapiche after so many years of absence led me to review the events of my early life in the forest and to think about their meaning. During these reflections I came to the conclusion that the present circumstances in which I lived made it impossible for me to train an apprentice by the methods I had been taught. The required isolation and rigor of training implied living off in the forest for more than a year, completely away from the disrupting influences that confront us when living in a civilized area. This of course was not possible to arrange, even assuming that I had a suitable candidate willing to undertake the training—which I did not. However, an alternative plan began to take shape in my mind. My fourth son, Roberto, finished secondary education not long after I returned from exile in Manaus. He was scholastically the brightest of my boys, and I thought if he could, by undertaking medical school training, obtain a license to practice medicine, we could then open a joint clinic. In this way there would be some hope and opportunity for passing on my knowledge of diagnosis and healing.

Roberto was enthusiastic about the prospect. In a few months he had passed entrance examinations and enrolled in pre-medical studies at Universidad Nacional de Trujillo. Everything went well for two or three years. But just as he became ready to enter medical school proper, the Peruvian Army closed the university down, claiming that it harbored a communist cell that was growing into a dangerous national influence. At that time the APRA party headed by Haya de la Torre was outlawed for communist leanings, and there was plenty of clandestine political agitation in Peru.

After months of controversy at the school where he hoped to return and complete his medical education, the situation became hopeless. He came to me one day in desperation, saying that he wanted to get married and start his family. What could I say? It was his life, and medical school no longer fit into it. And so I, for the second time, no longer had a suitable channel through which to assure the continuation of my healing methods.

My next assignment with Astoria after completing my botanical collection consisted of helping to organize the production of pharmaceutical materials already having a commercial market. These included *oje*[4] latex, *barbasco*[5] root from which the insecticide, rotenone, is extracted, and *curare*, the 'winged death' for which a surgical use as a muscle relaxant had been developed.

Insofar as my medical practice goes, *curare* is only a deadly poison. But I understand that doctors in North America and Europe purify the jungle extract, then synthesize fractions of it and do other things to it for all I know, so that they can use the final product as a precisely controlled muscle relaxant in certain delicate surgical operations. I have read that it has been used in cases of epileptic seizure to prevent bone fractures and to avoid bone deformations in poliomyelitis cases. There probably are many other uses. But the jungle extract containing a complex mixture of alkaloids seems recently to have been replaced by a simple synthetic product made in the chemical laboratory.

After my botanical collection was completed and sent off to New York one of the most important assignments with the company was organizing the production of commercial, medicinal-quality *curare* extract for export to New York. Many years ago as I have already described, I learned from old Izidoro of the Tikuna Indians on Ampiyacu Creek the secret of making this deadly arrow and blowgun-dart poison into a product that will not spoil. But the Indians mix many things, like scorpions, in their *curare* extract which makes it unsuitable for use in modern medicine.

The company developed a pharmaceutical market for *curare*, but then encountered difficulties with spoilage of the extract during its shipment to New York. Guillermo Klug, a German zoologist, who had been making the extract for the company at the beginning of the *curare* trade died, and a controversy developed over his death. From what the Tikuna Indians taught me about the extraction process and the properties of the product I think it was lack of care in making *curare* that caused Klug's death. We were good friends, so he confided in me about his production methods, and I know he was not careful enough about avoiding the fragrant vapors that arose from the pots during the boiling down of the extract to concentrate it for shipment.

When the product made by others less competent than Klug spoiled during transit, I was asked by the company to undertake the extraction of this product for which there was now a market that was not being supplied. The *ampihuasca* vine grows most abundantly in the forests on the foothills of the Andes in the country that I have already described for you. In the valley of the Rio Sisa in San Martín Province it grows as if it were planted, so that is where I went.

10

Curare from Rio Sisa

GOING UP INTO SAN MARTÍN AND THE RIO SISA COUNTRY FOR THE FIRST time, I began to understand why Juan Copete and Abelardo Torres who took me to Águano Isla were so desirous of returning from the flat, often-flooded country of the Rio Ucayali into the cool mountains. The Province of San Martín lies at the eastern foot of the Andes and is a wild mountainous country of steep ridges, narrow canyons, and cascading streams. Lush tropical vegetation covers everything except for a few rocky cliffs and bare ridges. Eyebrows of the mountains *(cejas de la montaña)* is a good name for it. A few narrow foot trails that the Lamisto Indians and their well-trained mules travel provide the only access to this incredible area.

Guillermo Klug had told me about his strange experiences working with the Lamisto. Because the men sent to continue the work after his death could not sustain a working relationship with them nor make an extract of satisfactory quality, *curare* production had come to a halt. But the demand for it from New York was urgent.

The small mountain village of Tarapoto in *curare* country is the main commercial center where the Lamisto trade. Here they bring coffee and other agricultural produce from their tiny mountain farm plots to barter for the few manufactured items they need. Near Tarapoto a ridgetop was found flat enough for an airport, and on my first flight there to investigate and plan *curare* production operations I carried letters of introduction to local traders who had dealings with the Lamisto. Tito Arévalo and Reinaldo Bartra tried to advise me on the difficulties of the country and the Indians when I arrived. But later experience showed me that they really knew very little of the wild country and the strange people I had to deal with. They did have trade relations with some of the Indians, but these connections were seldom and tenuous. I soon found the Lamisto to be superstitious and clannish people, and came to the conclusion that to get them to really work for me would require some more compelling motive than money.

As usual, luck was with me. Arévalo introduced me to Salas, a Lamisto from a small mountain village called Pamashto, and we got off to a good start when he found I could talk his brand of Quechua, common language of the mountain tribes. The Ecuadorian Santa Rosa Indians who had worked with me on the upper Tapiche had taught me Quechua and it came in very handy now.

Salas agreed to take me to San Pablo de Sisa off in the mountains where the last batches of unsatisfactory *curare* had been produced. We were two days on a mule trail that I thought would never come to an end. The first night we slept at a small hut hanging on the side of a mountain from which you could see several waterfalls through their rising clouds of mist, and in the distance off to the south a high spur range of the Andes called Blue Mountain was visible. Here the setting sun highlighted its topmost ridges in the gathering gloom of the main Andean shadow. Cold air drifting down from the snowy heights made us uncomfortable during the night even with a fire burning.

At Sisa the next afternoon I found the people very reserved and distant at first. Gradually with the help of Salas and my Santa Rosa Quechua we got a discussion of *curare* production going with some of the men who had gathered the *ampihuasca* vine for my predecessors. I soon learned that there were four varieties of the vine recognized by the Indians. They said no one had understood this before, but had mixed them all together and this had produced a poor extract.

Shortly I went out into the forest to collect a separate sample of these varieties, bringing back stem, leaves and flowers of each kind. With this material and using the deteriorating remnants of equipment that had been left there, I set out to make a separate sample of the extract from each variety. The Lamistos saw that I knew what I was doing, for of course I used the extraction method taught me by old Izidoro of the Tikuna Indian tribe whose *curare* was famous for its deadly strength all over the lower Amazon.

When my four samples were ready I returned to Tarapoto with Salas and sent the material by air to Iquitos, asking them to obtain an analysis of each as soon as possible and send me instructions on which variety of vine to use. The analysis, I knew, had to be done in New York and it would be several weeks before I could expect a reply.

While waiting I decided to have Salas show me where the best locations were for future *curare*-extraction camps. The vine was scattered in the mixed forest and a camp had to be moved each time the supply was exhausted in one area. I bought supplies at Tarapoto and we went on a mule trip from there to Pamashto, Salas' village, then on to Fausa Lamisto, Fausa Sapina, Saposoa, and down to Bella Vista on the Rio Huallaga.

At Bella Vista I paid Salas for the trip and sent him back to Pamashto, telling him I would send for him to come to Tarapoto as soon as I heard from Iquitos. On our excursion I had tried to gain his confidence and now felt that he would be helpful in my *curare* production efforts. From Bella Vista I flew back to Tarapoto on the first plane that made a stop there.

At Tarapoto I found a radiogram which read: *VARIEDAD AMARILLA NUMERO TRES MAXIMO CONTENIDO EXTRACTIVO FAVOR PRODUCIR DOSCIENTOS KILOS MAS PRONTO POSIBLE URGENTE* (YELLOW VARIETY NUMBER THREE MAXIMUM EXTRACTIVE CONTENT PLEASE PRODUCE AS SOON AS POSSIBLE TWO HUNDRED KILOS URGENT). There was also a letter with more detail, emphasizing that New York needed the *curare* extract, 200 kilos of it, as soon as I could produce it.

Arévalo and Bartra assisted in getting my supplies and equipment together and hiring the mules for transport. Luckily Ricardo Ramírez from San Pablo de Sisa was in Tarapoto on a trading trip and he helped me in the preparation and return trip to the *curare* camp near Sisa. It was a wild trip with a pack train of loaded mules, Ramírez taking the lead and I bringing up the rear.

Within a few days the Sisa *curare* camp was functioning. We found a clay bank along a small stream where we excavated a string of fireplaces, each with a kind of chimney over which the boiling pans could be placed. When a good supply of firewood was gathered

I sent the men out to cut the vine with instructions to bring in straight stems neither too old nor too young, and to cut only as much as they could bring in on one day so it would be fresh. Of course I made it clear I wanted only the yellow variety. And I had to keep a sharp eye on everything!

Ampihuasca is a large woody vine that hangs from the tree tops. The stem has a very irregular shape, full of indentations and cavities. Almost every vine is found to have scorpions hiding in these holes in the stem. Some of the men called the vine *madre del alacrán.* Every day I cautioned the men to give every vine section in their pack load a good pounding to dislodge this pest before they bound up the load to pack it to camp. Even so some of the men got scorpion stings on their shoulders or back.

In camp we cut the vine segments into ten-inch pieces. These were mashed by pounding them with a rock. Then we tied the mashed pieces with a small vine to hold the splinters together. Several of these bundles were put in the first large basin over the fire with plenty of water. As the water turned brown it was dipped into the next pan. More water and mashed vine were added to the first pan as needed. As the liquid got darker and more concentrated from evaporation of the water boiling away I dipped the liquid into other pans down the line, thus eliminating any sediment. The fire under the final pan had to be kept low and, as the whole batch of concentrate accumulated in that last pan, the liquid thickened. When it reached the point of becoming a stiff thread dripping from a dipper it was ready to go into the five-gallon tins where it solidified on cooling. If the fire burned too hot beneath the final pan at this critical stage of the process the batch would scorch and several days' work of the whole camp was lost.

Izidoro, the Tikuna Indian of Ampiyacu Creek, showed me this way of testing the *curare* with the dipper to find the proper point of removing it from the fire. I also learned first from him about the danger of inhaling the vapor from the cooking pans of *curare*. The steam turns your shirt yellow if you stand in the rising vapor. We always tried to choose a well-ventilated location for making the extract. I knew that sugar was a partial antidote for *curare* poisoning, so I kept a tin of hard candy in camp and passed some out every week or so to the men who helped in the boiling-down process.

In my first *curare* camp near San Pablo de Sisa, one day as we got a new batch of *curare* under way, I noticed that Ramírez' wife Concha, our camp cook, was talking strangely. I couldn't understand a thing she said. All of a sudden she had a spastic seizure and fell writhing into the cooking fire. Some of the men returning with firewood helped me get her out quickly before any harm occurred.

From watching her seizure I knew it was epilepsy. This bad omen meant that unless I could do something for her my days of *curare* production with the Lamistos were over. Ramírez told me afterward that she often had these seizures, but to have one in my *curare* production camp was nevertheless a bad sign for the project. In Iquitos I had cured a boy in carpentry school who had been in danger of injuring himself with sharp tools when epileptic fits came on him unexpectedly. I told Ramírez that I could probably cure his wife, and a look of amazement crossed his face.

I took out of my kit of medicines that I always carried with me when traveling a small piece of the liver-colored *pedernal*[1] (flint) rock from Pedernal Creek on the upper Rio Tapiche. Then I put a small pan on the fire to boil water. While the water heated I held the rock in the fire with a piece of wire. When the wire turned red I put the rock in the water and it shattered. I let this boil for several minutes, then removed the pieces of shattered stone and ground them into a fine powder. I mixed a spoonful of the powder and the water with the white of an egg and a pinch of powdered charcoal from the fire. This remedy I gave to Concha every morning for nine days as we went on with our *curare* production. Of course the effect did not show until time for her next seizure, but over the next several years that I worked off and on with Ramírez in the production of *curare* he told me she never had another seizure. He was very grateful and told all his friends that I had cured his wife.

In about three weeks I returned to Iquitos with the urgently requested *curare* concentrate. We boxed and shipped it to New York on the Booth Line and in a month or so a letter came back saying that the laboratory reported it was the best *curare* extract they had ever received. Also a request came for 500 kilos more produced in exactly the same way.

This time my friends in Tarapoto advised me when I returned that I was in danger of being robbed if I traveled the same route into my *curare* camp every time I came. Tito Arévalo suggested that I go the short distance down to Chazúta near the Rio Hullaga, then upstream to Bella Vista in a small boat with outboard motor, and from there to San Pablo de Sisa one day's mule trip back into the mountains. Arévalo told me he had one of the more reliable Chazutinos in town on a trading trip and perhaps we could persuade him to take me to Chazúta. When we talked to this man, named Chuquizuta, about taking me down to Chazúta and the Rio Huallaga, I could see that my use of his Quechua dialect caught his interest, and he had also heard about my curing Ramírez' wife of her fits, so he agreed to my returning with him to Chazúta.

Arévalo warned me, however, to be careful in dealing with the Chazutinos, saying that they were a superstitious bunch, committed to witchcraft, sorcery, and all kinds of wild spirits. But this seemed to me a situation I could turn to my advantage.

When we arrived at Chazúta it soon became clear to me that everything happening in the world around these people or among them was interpreted by them as emanating from some spirit source. This I realized was why they and their neighbors in the other Lamisto villages were so difficult to deal with. You could never tell what wild interpretations they would put on the commonest everyday event. But word of my driving the evil spirit out of Ramírez' wife had preceded me to Chazúta, and they told me they had a sick man dying of evil spirits. When I went to see him I found he was desperately ill all right, but more from the complications of malaria and intestinal parasites than from evil spirits.

To further improve my position I decided to stop and cure the man. I would need some of these people to work for me in the production of *curare*. The cure would take several days, and I would have to supervise it closely because I knew these superstitious Indians could not be trusted to follow my instructions if left to themselves. While in the forest gathering plants needed to prepare the extracts to treat the sick man I came upon the *ayahuasca* vine and the *yagé* shrub. I decided then to induce the Chazutinos to take the vision extract with me. There would be time while my patient recovered from his illness. So, in the forest a short distance from the village, I constructed a small palm-thatched shelter, gathered plants, and started the extraction process, first on those needed to cure my patient and then of the vision vine.

Taking my medicine, the man thought to be dying of evil spirits improved in a few days. During this time I selected a small group of men including Chuquizuta to take *ayahuasca* with me. I had found out in our long discussions that their experience with the vision vine was only superficial. With my comments on its true effects I aroused their curiosity to such a point that they became intrigued to see if what I said was true.

I have told you about taking *ayahuasca* with the men of Chazúta already. Those two vision sessions, it turned out, were of crucial importance to the success of my *curare* program. I had learned in long talks with some of the men, even before our first joint drinking of *ayahuasca*, that the large forest cats, the jaguars, were felt to be of special mystical importance to the Chazutino hunters. Some of them had even learned to trap this uncanny beast, hoping to find out more about him. It was because I knew the fascination the big cats held for these men that I led the visions so as to show them things which they would never forget. And from snatches of talk I heard afterwards, I knew they thought the jaguars of the forest were under my control and did my bidding.

By the end of our second vision session the ill *chazutino* whom I had been treating for malaria and parasites was recovered, and I had to get on with *curare* production. So in a day or so I moved on via Bella Vista to San Pablo de Sisa with Chuquizuta going along as helper.

In this small Lamisto village word of my coming had preceded me and Ramírez had selected a good place for the production camp. We all went to work and some of the men from Chazúta came along in a few days to help in the *curare* production.

When we were about halfway through with the production of the latest *curare* order, Ramírez' wife Concha came to me one day and said that one of the Chazutinos had stolen a large piece of salt fish from my supplies and had run off with it. I knew this meant trouble, especially if it were repeated. Several of the men were standing around and heard her accusation. Now I said in a loud voice, looking at Concha but knowing the men would hear me, "He will never enjoy that fish. A jaguar will get him before he has a chance!" Eyes rolled at this declaration, and I heard some whispering among the Chazutinos.

Ramírez sent one of his best San Pablo de Sisa trackers after the thief. Several days later he showed up in camp, exhausted and bedraggled. He told us that he had followed the thief up a narrow canyon high in the mountains. And he had finally come on the place where a jaguar had indeed attacked the man and carried him off up the canyon wall where it was impossible to follow.

Word of this spread like a gust of the wind, especially among the Chazutinos, who now were convinced beyond any doubt that I did of a certainty control the jaguars. Those big cats did my bidding! From that day on, I may say, nothing whatsoever was taken from camp without my permission.

The work of the *curare* production had to be coordinated with the style and manner in which the Lamisto lived. Theirs was a tight existence. Many of their farm plots were in inaccessible places where less vigorous people would not and could not go. The height of the rainy season and during harvest time toward the end of the dry season were both difficult times to try to recruit workers to bring in firewood and the sections of *ampihuasca* vine I had to have.

Their main yearly celebration was the fiesta of the Virgen del Carmen in August. At this time they would sing and dance for eight consecutive days, consuming at the same time prodigious quantities of food and home-made intoxicating beverages. To prepare for the fiesta several groups of five or six men would go off on hunting trips for as long as three months beforehand. They would hike off through the forest to the east across the Rio Huallaga toward the Rio Ucayali, and there would set up hunting camps and prepare smoked game. They called this *sacha aicha*, forest meat. Some of them even came out on the Rio Ucayali at Tierra Blanca and Sarayacu where they would trade for salt fish.

When the eight days of the celebration were over and they

wanted to sober up and recover, the women would make up great quantities of fish stew from salt fish, *yuca*, and hot peppers. This they called *paiche pango*—very nourishing and restoring food.

For several years I made at least two trips a year to work with my Lamisto friends in San Martín Province for the purpose of producing several hundred kilos of concentrated *curare* extract, all of which we sent to the New York pharmaceutical market. During that time Ramírez, Chuquizuta, and Isuisa were my most trusted Lamisto helpers. Occasionally, still, one of them sends word to find out how I am and when I plan to return to the Lamisto country of the Rio Sisa.

The last batch of *curare* extract that I made was finished in November of 1965, and I understand that the simpler synthetic preparation is now universally used. There no longer seems to be a market for the kind of *curare* the Lamisto and I produced from the forest vine.

Whenever I worked with the Lamisto, especially with the Chazúta group, I counselled them against the practice of sorcery and witchcraft. Telling them that this wickedness always resulted in bringing on attacks of vengeance and reprisal, I reminded them that it was always the practicing *brujo* or witch who suffers the ultimate assassination. Much better, I told them, to live at peace with your neighbors and die of old age, happy and tranquil among your family. Give up your witchcraft, I told them, or I will leave you, will banish you from my mind. From their reaction and from what I have heard I think they did heed what I said and gradually stopped practicing witchcraft on each other.

11

Arab Surgery

DURING THOSE YEARS WHEN I WENT REGULARLY TO SAN MARTÍN TO produce *curare* it would take about two months twice a year to supply the market. Mr. Allen on his annual visit from the New York office of Astoria would call me in to ask about the production of the *curare* and other plant extracts, and he would always give me advice on how to take care of myself in the forest. He would say "You must take good food and water with you. Don't eat the native food or drink the local water. It is dangerous. The company will pay for you to take care of yourself."

Little did he realize the actual working conditions in the forest. There were plenty of times when there was nothing but monkey stew or a bit of dried fish. Still, roast breast of jungle partridge once in a while made up for some of the less tasty menus.

Between times at the *curare* camps I carried out other assignments up and down the river. Somewhere on one of my river trips I vaguely remember eating a delicious fish stew and at the time felt that possibly a small fish bone had stopped somewhere along the way down my throat. The impression passed and I thought no more about it until one day soon after setting up a new *curare* camp in the mountains something I swallowed gave me a sharp pain about halfway down. By then there was nothing I could do. If I had gone to work on that fishbone when it first stopped in my throat I probably could have dislodged it, but not now.

What could I do? I had an urgent order for *curare* and must fill it as my employers expected. But each day my gullet became worse until I had to stop eating solid food, and toward the end I lived on the thinnest of broth which Concha fixed especially for me. The production of *curare* went on nevertheless. When the lot was finished several weeks later I could hardly get it to the airport at Tarapoto. If my relations with the Indians had not been good they would long since have stolen all my equipment and left me abandoned in the mountains. But this did not happen.

At Tarapoto my friends Arévalo and Bartra looked at me and shook their heads. I was crazy, they said, to have been staying in the mountains in my condition. And when I arrived at the office in Iquitos with the *curare* shipment the men hardly recognized me. One side of my head was all swelled up from the infection and the skin around my mouth was all peeling off. My lower jaw would not move and I had to talk through my teeth. I could hardly walk, I was so emaciated.

There was a big flurry of telephone calls and cablegrams. I was told to go to a local doctor the next morning for an examination. When I arrived at the clinic the doctor came, looked me over with a barely disguised expression of dismay on his face, and brusquely ordered me to open my mouth. By that time I could not speak, but I shook my head 'no,' seething at his improper approach to a patient. When the doctor came toward me with his hands raised as if he would force my mouth open, I turned on my heel and walked out of there.

Well, then there was more flurrying around, and that afternoon the company office manager showed me a cable from New York saying I should fly to New York for treatment at Company expense. I wrote on a piece of paper "No, Lima."

The next morning Nieves and I were on a flight over the Andes to Lima. We were met at the airport by my son who is an accountant for the Ministry of Public Health. And we went directly to the National Institute of Neoplastic Diseases. Doctors in Peru were calling everything cancer at that time so the government established this Institute to clarify the situation.

There was a good feeling about the place and my state of mind improved as soon as I stepped into the building. Of course, you know the first thing they do when you go into a hospital is to take your pants away from you so you can't get out. I was soon in bed with a bunch of pleasant-looking doctors around. They didn't try to open my mouth. My son by that time knew the story from Nieves and explained the development of my condition to the doctors.

I hadn't eaten or slept for days and was exhausted. Soon they had a bottle rigged up dripping liquid nourishment into a vein in my arm and I began to feel a little better. I went right to sleep and didn't wake up until the next morning.

The doctors came back, but only three now, two men and a woman. They did all kinds of tests including an x-ray, and I was becoming more alert after the good night's rest. Something in the liquid going into my vein was clearing up the inflammation on my face and around my mouth.

In two or three days they had me in pretty good shape. One of the doctors came to talk to me. I could tell he was an Arab by his color and demeanor. He told me he had heard about my knowledge and use of Indian medicines from the jungle, and said that their use was probably what had given me the resistance to stay alive. Then he explained that it would be a rather simple operation to remove the obstruction from my throat, to be done the next day.

That evening a little Spanish Padre came swishing in with his flowing black robes and lisping accent. Nieves was staying in the room with me but he paid no attention to her. "*Vosh queresh confeshar, mi hijsho*—You want to confess, my son?" he asked me.

Nieves told him firmly that I could not speak. That it was against the doctor's orders. But he persisted, asking me if when I was a boy I didn't steal things and chase girls.

There was a pad and pencil on the bedside table that I used to make notes to people. I picked up the pencil and wrote, "Yes, that was my main occupation. Now get out!"

"Ay, bendito," he said, shaking holy water all over the place. "*Diosh te bendigash*" (God forgive you) and he swished out the door with a flurry.

Nieves said something disrespectful and I tried not to smile because it hurt way down inside my throat.

The next morning about 9:30 an intern came in and gave me an injection, saying he would be back in half an hour. When he returned he seemed surprised that I had my eyes open. He said "Raise your hand if you hear and understand me" and I raised my hand.

Then he said "Raise your hand if you feel this" and he pinched my arm. I raised my hand again. He looked very confused, shook his head and went out.

Soon he was back with the Arab doctor. They gave me another injection and the doctor said, "That should put you to sleep." When they came back I was not asleep, and we went through the whole hand-raising performance again.

They went and came back shortly with two other doctors. Now they took my pulse, looked in my eyes, and solemnly shook their heads and talked about another injection. The Arab said to me, "We have never heard of a patient that didn't go completely to sleep on two injections of this anesthetic. But we are all ready upstairs for the operation and we will give you another. I nodded and they gave me the third injection, and left.

When they returned after a time I could still see, hear, and understand but could not raise my hand or move any part of my body so I closed my eyes to make them happy. And they wheeled me away on a silent cart. In the operating room I could understand everything they said and I think they realized it because they watched me and did not talk much. The woman doctor was French and she talked to the Arab doctor in French. But the other doctor was Italian and part of the talk had to be translated to him in Spanish which I could understand.

The French woman was an ear specialist, as I found out when they unhinged my lower jaw. She made them take great care so they would not damage my hearing. As soon as my jaw was unhinged the Italian pushed his hand up under my rib-cage from below until he had pushed the organs of my throat up into my mouth. Then the Arab cut out my fish bone with the tumor that had formed around it. It was all over in a few minutes, except for the sewing and placing the tubes through my nose to my stomach.

It was several hours before the numbing effect of the injections wore off—not until next day, actually. In a few days I could talk a little and the Arab came to ask me what jungle medicine I had taken that would cancel out his anesthetic injections. But I could not tell him.

When they took the stitches out of my throat this Arab

surgeon—his name was Ernesto Salem—told me he would come to Iquitos some day to sample some of my remedies. He never did come, which to me was a disappointment because I would have welcomed his closer scrutiny of the healing methods which I had developed. But I have seen him several times by chance on the streets of Lima. He always stops and shakes his head at me as he recalls his patient from the forest who would not go to sleep—even under a dose of anesthesia that would put most people away forever.

12

Rio Napo

MY FIRST TRIP TO THE RIO NAPO REGION DEVELOPED FROM THE EFFORTS of the Astoria Company to find a good place for a logging contractor to cut Spanish cedar for the company sawmill. Going up the Napo in the company launch we stopped at a place called Inayuga. Here I found the Mañanita and Irarica families who had formerly cut rubber for me on the Rio Blanco and Rio Tapiche. They had returned to their former home at Inayuga when the rubber trade completely collapsed shortly after I had moved from the Rio Tapiche to Águano Isla.

We had a big reunion when I found these people, and talked for a long time about all the things that had happened to us since those days on the Tapiche thirty years before. My friends were very helpful in giving me valuable information on the forests of the Rio Napo. They suggested that the best place to cut cedar trees was in the rich forests of the Rio Curaray, a tributary of the Napo above Inayuga. And after we had looked over the country, this was where the log contractor decided to locate. There on the Curaray he was a successful supplier of logs to the Astoria sawmill for a number of years. Later I helped develop other products which the company extracted from the forests of the Rio Napo.

José O'Neil, the manager of the Astoria Company operation in Iquitos, was an avid reader of books. And when Padre Avencio Villarejo's book *Asi Es La Selva*, written about the Amazon forest, appeared in Iquitos, Don José called me into his office for a discussion of its comments on medicinal plants and other products of the forest.

Padre Avencio had been traveling the rivers of the Peruvian

Amazon for many years. He was an astute observer of the people and the geography of the region, but as I pointed out to Don José, most of the information reported in his book was gathered by talking to people rather than from any firsthand experience in the forest. In my opinion this limited its value as a means of assisting us to find new commercial products that could be taken from the forest and promoted by the company. Nevertheless Don José insisted that I investigate two items mentioned by Padre Avencio, used, he said, by the people of the Rio Napo. One was *cupati*, a vine reportedly used by Indians for birth control, and the other, *yoco*[1], a plant from which a stimulant is extracted that prevents fatigue.

This was in the 1950's when the company was very much interested in taking advantage of the pharmaceutical search for commercial contraceptive substances. I had knowledge of several plants used by various Indian tribes, but that is something I will tell you about later because it does not involve the Rio Napo. As it turned out *cupati* proved worthless as a practical commercial product.

The investigation of *yoco* turned out to be an interesting enterprise but it also failed to produce anything marketable. My Mañanita Indian friends at Inayuga told me I could find *yoco* in the territory of the Secoya Indians that lived on Santa Maria Creek up near the Ecuadorian border. When I found out that Roque Guerrero of Camp Serio traded with the Secoya I asked him to go with me to one of their villages.

Here on Santa Maria Creek, also called Secoya Creek, there were two villages. *Curaca* Santos, Chief Santos, at that time led the clan called the Angutieros or Peaceful Ones. The Saparos or Smart Ones were a clan living further up the creek.

I worked mostly with Santos and his people. Their Secoya language is very difficult to pronounce and understand, but they know Quechua also and we had no real trouble understanding one another. Compared to the Lamisto, working with the Secoya was easy. While I stayed with them Chief Santos provided me with food and a small house. He was the *curandero*, the healer, for the tribe and we exchanged information about the medicinal properties of the plants in his area.

But the Secoya were also a superstitious people, their complicated beliefs almost incomprehensible. They believed that most of their troubles came from some *brujo* (witchdoctor) with stronger power than their own casting an evil spell on the victim. Their use of medicinal plants for curing was rather simple. The usual practice was for Chief Santos to sing, suck out thorns, blow smoke onto the affected part of the body, sometimes while massaging—all to little effect in my opinion. But the belief in witchcraft caught up with Chief Santos. I heard only recently that when a woman died in the village of the Saparo, the villagers were convinced it was by Santos' witchcraft. In revenge they assassinated him. A great pity, but I was not among them long enough to change their beliefs.

Neither Santos nor any of the other Indians with whom I have worked since leaving the Huni Kui possess the complete knowledge of the forest plants displayed by my former captors. It seems to me as I have thought about this difference many times that the advantage held by the Huni Kui came from the more complete domination and control of the reactions in the mind brought about by taking *ayahuasca*, the vision-vine drink.

The Secoya, and most of the other Indians I worked with except of course for the Huni Kui, used only a cold water extract of the vine without adding the leaves of the shrub *chacruna* or *yagé*. Taking this cold water infusion has a much less profound action on the mind than the boiled extract, from my experience, and thus gives those who use it a much shallower understanding of their environment. Regardless of this, I learned some valuable things about the forest of the Rio Napo from Chief Santo and his people there on Secoya Creek.

They showed me without hesitation the woody forest vine called *yoco* and how it is used. The bark is scraped or grated into cold water and allowed to settle. The water when poured off has a cloudy, sometimes a brownish, look. These Indians when they have a phyically difficult job to do or a long trip to make overland drink a small cup of *yoco* before starting. It gives them stamina to carry out extraordinarily difficult work that would leave most men exhausted. I have taken it with them before going on long hunting trips in the forest and can testify from firsthand experience that it works. And there are no undesirable after-effects from taking *yoco*, at least so far as I could determine.

I sent an ample shipment of material from this vine to New York for testing. When the report came back it stated that *yoco* had a high content of the alkaloid caffeine and nothing more of interest, so the investigation was dropped. But somehow I feel that there is more to *yoco* than this because of the physical reactions I myself have tested. You can get a bad set of coffee nerves from drinking too much black coffee. *Yoco* does not produce this reaction, and I think therefore the alkaloid must differ somehow from caffeine.

One day when we were off in the forest gathering *yoco* for my sample shipment I noticed Santos looking at my arm with a frown. He pointed to a small red-headed fly standing on its head biting me. He slapped my arm and mashed the fly, then stood shaking his head. "*Uta*,"[2] he said, "that fly causes *uta*, very bad. It will not show up for many months and may not show up at all, but that fly carries the disease *uta*. You know what that is?"

To make certain of the malady and its vector, I asked him "You mean the bite of that fly causes the dreaded skin ulcer that usually appears on the shin bone, but also invades the cartilage of the nose and ears, causing grotesque disfiguration? And finally nose and ears may drop off?" With a deep frown and worried look on his face, Chief Santos nodded, but looked relieved when I told him that I knew of a cure.

Six months later on a trip up the Rio Tapiche I did indeed begin to experience the symptoms of *uta*. Soreness, swelling, and inflammation began to develop in my neck just below one ear, along with an itching spot on one shin. The ear also became inflamed. These symptoms I recognized, but as I had told Santos, I also knew the cure. From the forest I gathered the roots of a vine called *rumosarsa,*[3] a relative of the better known *sarsaparilla*. Boiling these roots in water with brown sugar, I made a thick *jarabe* or syrup. After taking this syrup three times a day for several weeks the soreness and the beginning ulcers of *uta* disappeared, along with the inflammation in my neck and ear. As you see, I avoided the usual permanent disfiguring of my nose and ears.

In addition to *yoco* the Secoya have a vine called *macote*[4]. They use this interesting plant as a fish poison in bodies of still water, such as lakes and lagoons or bayous. The Indians gather this woody vine from the forest and mash it by pounding it with a rock or heavy wooden club. In the evening they make two canoe trips across the water which they wish to poison, scattering the *macote* on the water. In the morning they return to gather up the fish and anything else they might want from what lived in that water. This *macote* vine kills everything, including turtles and alligators; it also kills the anaconda, the big water boa. I have seen the Capanahua Indians on the Rio Tapiche use this vine, too. It seemed to me that this poison should be of some interest to science because it is more effective in killing aquatic life than *barbasco* which yields the rotenone for commercial insecticides. However, there was no reaction from the sample sent to New York for analysis.

After my first trip to the Secoya, about 1954, *ojé*[5] latex and rosewood oil extraction became important activities that took my time on the Rio Napo and in other locations. From the tree of the fig family called *ojé* there is extracted a free-flowing latex with important medicinal properties. Chemical analysis has shown that this latex contains an anthelmintic enzyme named *ficina*. As with *curare* I found that there are several varieties of *ojé*, some of which have a higher content of the desired enzyme than others. One of the best is a small leaf variety called *shiquaco ojé* found in the Rio Napo forests. I spent many months in those forests organizing and instructing various groups in the best method of producing *ojé* latex.

I had an interesting experience with *ojé* in Iquitos. Several of my grandchildren go to the Iquitos schools and for this reason I was prevailed upon to act for a time as president of the parent-teacher association. During this tenure the director of the school system came to me one day and said he needed to consult with me about a school medical problem.

I replied, "Of course. I am at your service. Perhaps that is a field where I am qualified to give advice. What is the problem?"

"We have received a number of complaints from parents who say their children are coming home from school bloated. And at least one child has become seriously ill. I am not sure of the cause but I wonder if it may be from our attempt to combat intestinal parasites in our pupils. You know that one of the principal medical problems of school age children in this area is intestinal worms."

"Yes, but that is a complicated problem, not for the schools to solve without competent medical advice. What have you been doing about this?" I asked.

"Well, Don Manuel, as you know, the standard home remedy of the Cocama Indians for this problem is to use the latex extracted from the *ojé* tree and many people have adopted this remedy. My own mother used it on us when we were kids. Now you know the drugstores have a commercial preparation of this, easy to use. You don't have to go to the forest for the *ojé* latex anymore. This is called Padax and comes in small packets of yellowish powder. I am sure you know of it. We have been giving doses of Padax to children in some of our schools."

He must have read the look on my face, because the Director of Schools got rather nervous at this point.

"You don't remember the diet your mother put you on when you took *ojé*?" I asked him. "You are very lucky if you have not had any serious medical complications among your students. Diet is the most important part of the *ojé* or Padax treatment, and this crucial part is beyond the control of the school. However well-intentioned your people may be, ridding your students of intestinal parasites is outside the province of education and they are on very treacherous ground should serious complications show up.

"You do not find me, a healer, entering into the field of education. And I recommend in the strongest terms possible that you stop practicing medicine in your schools unless you have competent medical advice. It is absolutely ridiculous to give students Padax without medical supervision. Luck is with you if you have avoided lawsuits. You had better call your schools at once and insist that no more Padax be distributed."

My visitor thanked me and departed, and the schools stopped distributing Padax powder to their pupils. So far as I have heard there have been no complications.

The Cocama Indians who live in the same river bank environment as the *ojé* tree have no doubt used *ojé* latex for generations as a remedy for intestinal worms. I have known and worked with many Cocama families. They are a healthy and robust people even in their difficult environment. But they do not maintain their health by using carelessly the natural remedies which they have learned to take to counteract their diseases.

When a purge for intestinal parasites is needed—and they know the symptoms—a time is chosen when the individual will not have to be doing much work but can remain quiet. The old Cocama *curandero* carefully chooses a young *ojé* tree that is free of either flowers or fruit. From a cut in the bark he obtains a large bottle of latex. This is mixed with an equal amount of fresh sugar-cane juice in a glass jug. Then he puts this mixture aside to ferment for eight days. The Indian taking the treatment begins his day without eating anything; he picks a comfortable spot, sits down, and calmly, little by little, drinks the whole jug of the fermented *ojé* mixture. The result is a mild but absolutely thorough purge of the intestinal tract. And the Cocama has learned that what he eats following the purge is very important. For a whole week his food is restricted to boiled but unsalted rice and unsalted smoked fish. He knows it is especially important not to eat sugar or anything sweet for at least three weeks. Then he gradually goes back to his normal diet.

You will never see an anemic or rickety Cocama Indian and this treatment is the reason. But these natural remedies are dangerous if improperly prepared, or if they are used, without adequate observation and control, by someone who does not know what he is doing. I do not myself use the *ojé* cure for intestinal parasites anymore, because of the difficulty of controlling the patient's diet. There are less complicated remedies for eliminating these parasites.

13

El Botanico

One day in the course of our 1961 forest survey as we were returning through the forest to our motor launch Córdova stopped along a low ridge of ground barely a foot above the surrounding swamp water. He pulled up a small woody shrub and beat the roots gently against a tree trunk to get rid of the dirt, then examined both the leaves and the root. "*Sanango*,"[1] he said, "good medicine, purifies the blood." When we got back to the launch he wedged the plant up under a roof support to dry in the shade.

Thus, from many small daily incidents during those months we spent together in the tropical jungles of the Peruvian Amazon I gradually became aware of my companion's commitment to medicinal plants from among the vast and myriad flora. The *sanango* incident occurred when we were surveying the forest along the Rio Samiria, a meandering, black-water stream that drains a large expanse of swamp between the Rios Marañon and Ucayali. It was on that trip that Córdova first told me about his botanical collection.

By this time we had been together constantly for several months and we recognized our mutual interests in the forest and its inhabitants. While navigating upriver on our launch, the Chontaquiro, to our next point of penetration into the forest, Córdova told me about the work he had done when he returned to Peru from his exile in Brazil.

"Before leaving Manaus I was told that Astoria wanted me to assist in investigating the commercial use of medicinal plants of the forest. When I got back and reported to work there in Iquitos, they gave me instructions on how to prepare botanical specimens and told me to make a complete collection of all the medicinal plants that I knew—including leaf, flower, fruit, bark and root of each plant.

"You know," he said, "it has been ten years since I completed that assignment and nothing has been said about the results. The company is changing now and I wonder what happened to my plants. It took me two years, mostly up the Rio Tapiche, to make the collection. There were two large wooden cases containing over a hundred specimens carefully prepared and sent to New York, with a report on how the plants were used. They told me my plants would then be scientifically identified, analyzed, and the results published for the benefit of medical science in Peru."

By this time I was very much intrigued by Mr. Córdova and his knowledge of the forest flora and fauna. I found that he could identify the slightest sound or scent of the jungle and could interpret many forest events that my sense receptors could not even detect. So I told him, "Look, when I go back to New York I will try to find out what happened to your plants. If we can find the collection and the botanical identification of the individual plants, then you and I can collaborate on the publication of a paper about their origin and use."

He was enthusiastic about this, but we had an extensive forest survey to complete before we could give more thought or effort to our possible scientific and literary collaborations.

Several months later when I had left the exotic smells, sounds, and vistas of the Amazon forest far behind and was traversing the asphalt jungles and granite canyons of New York City, I made inquiries about Mr. Córdova's botanical collections at the home office of his company. Don Manuel had been right when he said his company was changing. I was told by the first person I asked not to expect too much, that the man in charge of the Peruvian operations had retired an alcoholic. Then I was referred to the man in charge at present. He repeated the earlier comment, saying it was his impression that the botanical material had been sent out to various pharmaceutical companies without even proper records being kept of where the individual items had gone. But he suggested I return a week later; they would search the files and storage area to see what could be found.

When I came back I was given a pitifully small bundle wrapped in brown paper and told this was all that could be found, except for a typed report[2] with Córdova's name on it. The report gave the common, local names for the plants and their uses. In its margin was a handwritten key number tying each name and plant description to the corresponding specimen in the botanical collection. Don Manuel had certainly carried out his part of the bargain. This company executive suggested I take the small package of plants to the New York Botanical Garden for identification; perhaps at the Garden further light could be shed on the rest of the collection. And he gave me a letter of introduction to a botanist there who was working with Amazon plants.

Several days later at the Botanical Garden the package of plant material was unwrapped and the dried specimens examined. Obviously these consisted of mere remnants from material that had been picked over and divided up. From this incomplete material only the most tentative and partial identification could be made, and when I asked if the Botanical Garden had participated in the identification of the original complete collection, the botanist answered firmly, "No."

This brought to a dead end the correlation of Mr. Córdova's esoteric knowledge of Amazon flora with the botanical and medical science of the world. Botanical identification and taxonomic classification of plants is essential to the verification of Don Manuel's use of plant materials in healing and to the further development of this use in the interest of the health of mankind.

An easy reaction is to say "so what?" But as a young Peruvian jounalist wrote in the *Revista Trinchera*[3] after interviewing Don Manuel following the publication of *Wizard of the Upper Amazon,** *"Pero ahí están las cartas testimoniales, allí están los 500 pacientes que busca cada mes las pocimas contenidas en botellitas que entrega don Manuel. ¿Quien sabe si allí puede estar nadando un próximo milagro contra el cancer?"* ("But here are testimonial letters; there are the 500 patients who seek every month the potions con-

* *Wizard of the Upper Amazon: The Story of Manuel Córdova-Rios* by F. Bruce Lamb, Houghton Mifflin Company, 1975.

tained in the little bottles given out by Don Manuel. Who knows if the next miracle against cancer may be swimming there?'')

Ten long years passed after I promised to trace Don Manuel's botanical collections before I felt the situation was right for me to tell him the sad result of my search. His reaction was remarkable and definitely different from my own, which had been dismay and disgust. The time inevitably came one day when I tried to get from him a better description of a plant used in a special cure, and he said to me, ''That plant was in the collection I sent to New York. You can find out about it there.'' Then I had to tell him about my fruitless quest for his plants, and the reason for my searching questions now. When I had finished telling him the whole unhappy story he paused for a moment, seemingly in deep thought before he made any response.

''*Amigo*, I understand the disappointment you show in telling me of your findings. Perhaps you think I should be boiling over with anger. On the contrary, after all the good things the company and its people did for me in making possible my return from exile and later during my employment, my feeling is still more of gratitude than rancor.

''A good example is that of Don José O'Neil, the Astoria manager. He was an educated man, a lawyer, and observant of the people who worked for him. One day he called me in and said, 'Manuel, you have a great gift of healing, but you could increase your understanding and effectiveness by study, especially of human anatomy.'

''He gave me a large volume on anatomy written in Spanish, and this was only the beginning. When I returned a book he would give me another and would encourage me to continue my studies. One of the most helpful was a Spanish translation of a Japanese series called *Practical Medicine* from the Institute Arima Inagy of Botanical Sciences in Osaka, Japan. These studies brought to the conscious level of my mind and verified the knowledge that I had been using instinctively from the unconscious mind, retrieved through the use of *ayahuasca*. This gave me increased confidence in my methods of diagnosis and use of natural plant substances in healing. There seems to be a lot in common between my method of healing and that developed in the Orient using natural plants for treatment of illness. I understand that Japanese practices lean heavily on traditional Chinese healing techniques. I have had contact with American botanists and pharmaceutical investigators also, but in the final analysis it seems to me that we have very little in common. They always seem to expect me to tell them everything I know, show them all the plants I use, but nothing ever comes back in exchange.

"The company has asked me to work with several botanists from the Field Museum in Chicago, the New York Botanical Garden, and others I do not remember. All of these I have helped find notable plants they were looking for or discover new plants, none of which they would have found or recognized without my assistance and knowledge. One botanist I remember came looking for a plant he called 'Clusia' that had been collected and written about by a German botanist back in the 1800's. This plant had been lost to science ever since in spite of intense botanical search. When the plant was described to me I took this American botanist to a place where it grows profusely. He became so excited over his find that he drank a little too much that evening in a nearby mountain town and started giving money away to the Indian children on the street.

"Another time, it was in the mid-1950's during the search for the birth control pill, Mr. O'Neil asked me if I knew of plants that would limit human fertility. I told him of course I did; most Indian tribes use such substances. In a few weeks word arrived that a botanist was coming to work with me to study these plants."

Córdova went to his desk then and pulled out a file folder. Leafing through the papers, he handed me a faded newspaper clipping from a Lima paper, *La Prensa*, dateline Iquitos.

> J.B. Thiersch, doctor of pharmacology from the University of Washington, is in this city to study a series of medicinal plants that are used by the people of the Selva.
>
> The studies of Dr. Theirsch are entirely specialized and the results will not be known sooner than three years; for according to our informant, the process

> of reaction is delayed in the experiments that will be carried out on each plant.
>
> A small laboratory has been installed in one of the departments of Astoria Importing on the bank of the Rio Nanay. This will be the work center for the visiting scientist. Dr. Thiersch will be in Iquitos for a month more or less and then will return to the U.S. where the studies mentioned will be carried out.
>
> "It is impossible to anticipate the results of the studies I am beginning. Therefore I don't know whether the conclusions I will arrive at will be positive or negative," said Dr. Theirsch.

As I handed the clipping back to Córdova, he said, "When the doctor came we flew in a small pontoon plane to the Army Post at Chanchalagua on the Rio Tapiche. From there Jorge Pereira took us in a small boat with outboard motor several days farther upriver to where the highland forest starts, near where the homes of the first Capanahua Indians used to be on the river. There we made camp and went a half hour back into the forest to find the plants I thought Dr. Thiersch should test for contraceptive properties. We gathered material from two forest vines—leaves, stem and root. One was *abutilla,*[4] the other *gayo*[5] or *tumbo*. This material was packaged so that it would not dry out and we hurried back to Chanchalagua to be picked up by the plane for the return to Iquitos. When we got back to Iquitos it took us a week to make the extracts from those plants, working night and day in the lab we set up at Nanay. These extracts were put into five-gallon glass carboys for shipment to the testing laboratories in the United States. And that was the end of my involvement."

Of course I wanted to know more, and I said, "Don Manuel, this all happened several years ago. What report did you get on the results?"

Throwing up his arms and grunting with disgust, Córdova continued with his story, "Word finally came back that the extracts did not work on rats, so the tests were a failure. What can you do with such people? I didn't tell the doctor that the extracts would work on rats! I've never used them on rats! But I've used them on people, including my own daughter, and I know they work! Of course it is always possible that I did not get back the real answer. Dr. Thiersch never sent any word.

"But returning to my daughter—it turns out she grew up a bit wayward in spite of anything we could do. After she gave birth to the second child 'from the street' as they say in Iquitos, both of which my wife had to take care of, Nieves insisted that I had to do something to change things before she had another infant to care for.

"We called my daughter in and explained to her how intolerable the situation had become for us. I told her that if she would follow my instructions I could, without any ill effect on her health, make it so that she would not become pregnant again. It was no big scene. She was reasonable about it and I prepared the plant extracts for her treatment the same as I did for Dr. Theirsch's studies, and made certain that she took them as I instructed. It has been many years now, and my daughter is happily married, satisfied with the two children that Nieves took care of for her, and has had no more since taking the plant extracts I prepared for her.

"As I said before, I never tried this on rats, but it works on people. What do you suppose they really did with the material we sent for experimentation?

"It seems the scientists that come to explore the properties of the Amazon flora become famous for their discoveries. But few if any of them mention the contribution of their local collaborators. And yet people who come to pick my brains now wonder why I tell them so little.

"Recently professors of psychiatry and others have come over the mountains from the University of San Marcos in Lima seeking information on my power to control the reaction from taking the much sought-after *ayahuasca*. When I have told them that the famous vine has many secret properties that will cause them harm before they really discover anything of interest they generally leave me alone. I always try to avoid giving anything to these *buscavidas* (freeloaders), for when something of value results *they* always become the great discoverers of the material from the Amazon *selva* that will help humanity without any mention of me as the source. This has already happened to me several times.

"For some time now these people have been seeking *ayahuasca* preparations to test in Lima. But the results apparently have been negative because the extracts are prepared by people with little knowledge and responsibility, who will take advantage of anyone if they can. These investigators seem to think that with tape recorders, flash bulbs, and cameras they will be able to record some marvel from *ayahuasca* vision sessions organized among unprepared people, using improperly made vine extract. But they are mistaken. The secrets are not so easily available.

"Just recently a Dr. Picon from Lima has been here to study the case of *ayahuasca*. He will die of old age before he finds out anything worthwhile, the way he is going at it. For some reason these psychiatrists, Dr. Picon among them, think that they can cure mental disorders with *ayahuasca*. That is not so. But the Huni Kui know a tree they call *shatanapo*, and baths made from an extract of the tree bark will relieve mental unbalance. With *shatanapo* tree bark and the mineral extracted from the *pedernal* stone of the Capanahua I have cured several manic-depressives who wanted to commit suicide. *Ayahuasca*, it tells you how, but by itself it cures nothing directly."

Manuel Córdova's reaction to his encounters with visiting scientists seems to me revealing of at least one of the shortcomings of the scientific method[6] and the viewpoint of its practitioners in coming to grips with the resources of the Amazon region. The practice of orthodox scientific analysis results in dividing large problems into smaller and smaller segments to achieve simplification and control in the interest only of obtaining experimental results that are understandable, manageable, and repeatable. From the application of this scientific method have come technological developments that dazzle the mind. But there is now a growing awareness of the ill effects that inevitably result from the uncoordinated application of technology based on over-simplified analyses. Serious environmental degradation is the price we pay for technological developments which lack integration with the complex operations of nature. The relatively new discipline of ecology—with its stress on the interrelatedness of all natural systems—provides a scientific framework for judging and correcting at least some of the negative aspects of technology.

The tropical forest ecosystems of the Amazon are probably the most complicated in the world. The systematic dividing of these biological complexes into small segments for analysis has hardly begun, much less the process of putting the pieces back together to determine how they function. The scientists with whom Córdova has had contact have been so preoccupied with trying to understand their own little professional segments of Amazonian complexity that the two—Córdova and his protagonists—seem to have had little common ground for understanding each other. These scientists suspect the validity of Córdova's knowledge since it has not been derived from the rigors of scientific analysis and conventional scientific dogma. He considers their approach to understanding so narrow and shallow as to be almost without meaning. This dichotomy, it seems to me, is unfortunate and has already resulted in the loss of much useful knowledge, including the plant collections of Manuel Córdova which, if they had been taxonomically identified and analyzed, could have opened up whole new vistas in the art of healing.

Elizabeth Janeway,[7] author and critic, writing in *The New York Times Book Review* recently, said: "It is extremely difficult for modern men, including most modern scientists, to imagine that our 'primitive' ancestors [including primitives today] were not dreaming children. This is a failure of our imagination . . . we are prisoners of the present . . . we lose the power to believe in the effectiveness of other systems of knowledge . . . we confuse other conceptual structures with magic and the occult . . . [but] when science seems to be failing, we still call in the shamans."

This confusion between categories of thought and purpose impedes any progress in mankind's on-going adaptation to the complex and varied habitats on our planet. The principal hope for the future comes from expanding interest in integrative sciences and disciplines like ecology which work to sharpen our perception and raise our consciousness of the interrelatedness of all things, animate and inanimate.

I had already learned, long before I met Don Manuel, to respect the complexities of intricate tropical forest ecosystems, first in the jungles of Trinidad in the West Indies and then in such diverse locales as Guatemala, Borneo, West Africa, and the Amazon forest itself. My training and experience in interpretive forest analysis may have prepared me to view the events of Manuel Córdova's life from an unusual perspective, picking up clues of authenticity unheeded by others. There is an important message woven into the spell cast in his being by the *ayahuasca*. Perhaps, like his wife Doña Nieves, I have received something of his visions without partaking of the extract myself. If viewed only from the vantage point of forest ecology the accommodation Córdova had made to the Amazon environment and his accomplishments in this difficult realm carry an important message that should not be ignored. On the other hand I am well aware that there are those who consider him little more than a spinner of windy stories. As a matter of fact, one anthropologist, Robert L. Carneiro of the American Museum of Natural History in New York, has, on the basis of information not pertinent to the situation and time frame in question (in my opinion), attempted to cast doubt on the authenticity of the experience basic to Córdova's knowledge, recounted in the book *Wizard of the Upper Amazon*. Carlos A. Seguin, former Director of the Institute of Social Psychiatry, National University of San Marcos in Lima, Peru, joined in challenging Córdova's veracity by quoting Córdova himself in a letter to Carneiro. The line in question comes from an interview with San Marcos University staff and others given in the last year of Córdova's life, 1978, when he was 90 years old.

This provocative statement, *"No crean todo lo que les digo. Puede ser todo mentira,"* is susceptible to numerous different translations, especially if taken out of context. Córdova's daughter Adela accompanied him to the interview and in January 1979 in Iquitos she described the event to me. She considered her father's discourse remarkable in the light of his advanced age and poor health. Considering what Adela told me about the interview, I would translate the quotation given above as: "It might be misleading if you take literally all that I tell you." Carneiro translated this from Seguin's letter as: "Don't believe everything I tell you. It could all be a lie."[8] Córdova did realize the unique nature of his experiences and did say to me on several occasions during our long association *"Espero que usted no vaya a considerar que estas experiencias raras solamente vienen de la imaginacíon de un charlatan* (I hope you will not consider that these strange experiences come only from a charlatan's imagination)." He gave no intimation, however, that his revelations were less than truthful.

Manuel Córdova on his 91st birthday, November 22, 1978, passed on to other spheres of reality, and therefore cannot answer these criticisms of his commentary on life in the Peruvian Amazon forest.[9]

14

Uncanny Knowledge

My rapport and empathy with Córdova came from our mutual interest in the tropical forest ambience, from sharing his experiences with such people as the men of Chazúta, Izidoro of the Tikuna, the Inucuini, the Capanahua, and Chief Santos of the Secoya around our campfires. But often I wonder what strange, esoteric knowledge has escaped my understanding by not taking *ayahuasca* with Don Manuel. This did not result from reluctance on my part. Really there never was a situation when the surrounding conditions came up to Córdova's specifications. By the time we worked together he no longer required visionary stimulus to achieve his purpose, and therefore he did not have the extract readily available. Perhaps the nearest we came to taking the vision vine extract together was at Santa Elena on the Rio Tigre. But Córdova would neither partake himself nor permit me to imbibe of such poorly prepared *ayahuasca*. He understood too well the dangers of being ill prepared for the powerful release from this stimulant, even worse if it were improperly extracted from the vine.

On one of my occasional visits to Iquitos, several years after our timber survey had been completed, I decided to pursue the matter. We were seated in comfortable cane chairs in a cool breezeway of Córdova's home. I had not seen him for over two years, and was determined to eliminate some of the obscurity surrounding his rare capacity to diagnose human ailments and his ability to develop effective cures.

Discussing these matters with Don Manuel in his home inevitably became a more formal affair than the earlier explorations of our mutual interests in the forest. The contrast led me to recall the setting of our earlier discussions. Working side by side in the jungle I had been constantly reminded of Córdova's tremendous physique for a man then in his late seventies. Giving each other a hand over the obstacles of some rough terrain I had occasionally grabbed him by the upper arm and felt muscles as hard as rock, not a flabby fiber in his body. He could walk into exhaustion anyone in our timber survey party when we were in the forest. Not a giant by Corn Belt or professional football standards, he was a solid, compact man whose presence stood out in any group. Sitting in repose, smoking his ever-present pipe and conversing quietly, he gave the impression of a benign presence. His dark brown eyes in an impassive face took on an animated, penetrating glitter when any discussion included his jungle experiences or medical practice. An entertaining conversationalist, Córdova mimicked in voice and imitated in gesture the characters in his varied anecdotes drawn from a long adventurous life.

Little known outside his own country, Córdova was a famous *curandero-ayahuasquero*, a visionary healer, in Peru, especially in his own Amazon territory east of the Andes. Off and on over the years in both brief and more extended encounters I have attempted to grasp the elusive quality of this extraordinary man, the mystery in him, but our modes of thought and expression were basically worlds apart. Even though Don Manuel was obviously anxious to cooperate, adequate understanding between us seemed to require some additional frame of reference I groped for but had not yet found. Now in renewed pursuit of that common ground of understanding, I sought to explore the role and effect of taking *ayahuasca*, as I reminded him of our brief adventure on the banks of the Rio Tigre.

"Do you remember when we came on those two Indians preparing to take *ayahuasca* at Santa Elena on the Rio Tigre?"

"Yes, of course," he replied, "but that has been a few years ago now."

"Those two Indians there at Santa Elena whom you talked to in some strange tongue I could not understand, Don Manuel . . . you said they told you they were going to brew a batch of *ayahuasca* and drink it that night to discover the malady and cure for the sickness one of them suffered. Just how would all this appear to them in their visions there at night in that forest hut on the bank of the river?"

"We have discussed these things before, *amigo*," Don Manuel said to me, "and you know how difficult it is to explain what goes on in one's mind under the influence of *ayahuasca*.

"You remember I had some reservations about the inadequate care they were taking with their preparation of the extract—with a small boy boiling it in an old, dirty, beat-up aluminum kettle. But assuming the extract turned out to be suitable and that they took it by proper dosage in a setting of complete tranquility, and if they had the experience and understanding required to control the progress of the resulting visions, then—but only then—the source of the sickness in the body would have been revealed to them in detail. In addition, the plants required for the cure and how they should be prepared would also appear to them in the visions."

"But Don Manuel, what is the source of this knowledge?"

"For myself, the source is the songs or chants that I learned over fifty years ago during my training with old Chief Xumu of the Huni Kui, before he died. The progression of the visions is influenced, or controlled, by the chants and songs."

"And the chants?" I persisted, "Where did they come from; where did this accompanying knowledge come from, my friend?"

"*Compañero*, you are leading me in a circle, or perhaps it is a spiral. This knowledge had to come from tribal traditions accumulated and handed down for generations. And it seems to me that those Indians I lived with were tapping biological memories, some deeply buried memories of the race, stemming from who knows what source and what time. Their belief was that the animals now and in the past taught them in visions the secrets of the forest they needed to know."

Córdova then went deeper into this subject.

THE BEGINNING OF EVERYTHING FOR ME IS—*EL ORIGEN DE TODO ESTO POR mi parte es un afluyente de energia, suave y armonioso de la inconsciencia profunda*—a continuous smooth and harmonious flow of energy from deep in the unconscious. But to achieve the consonant flow through the nervous system you must avoid an initial violent and disruptive discharge of energy that often occurs at the beginning. To control the power which reveals the secrets of *ayahuasca* requires preparation and training.

I have described for you the lengthy, difficult, and sometimes frightening apprenticeship I went through in my youth with old Chief Xumu. You remember that for my first participation in a group vision session with the Huni Kui, Xumu kept me on a carefully controlled diet for several weeks and gave me purging plant extracts to drink, along with special herbal baths. During the year or more of intensive apprenticeship that followed I was given only certain foods and compelled at critical times to abstain from all physical exertion, including sexual activity with the girls the chief had given to me. And during the actual visions I had the constant tutelage of a Master using who knows how many generations of tribal knowledge and experience to control my progress.

The old chief and the others of the tribe emphasized by word and act at every opportunity that I was to be their tribal healer. Each one of them attempted to transfer his individual knowledge of plants to me both during vision sessions and afterward when we were in the forest together. With the heightened sense perception that came from taking the extract of the vision vine, I was able to observe and perceive qualities of plants entirely obscure to the unprepared observer.

Altogether during those years I spent with the Huni Kui I must have been initiated through *ayahuasca* over 500 times. On each occasion it was taken only after several days of rigorous dieting, and during the early training stages all this was under the careful vigilance of the Chief. After he died I had several years more with the Indians to use, amplify and perfect my healing practices. I received from the Huni Kui a true transmission of how the vision vine reacts, and I learned to manage my reactions as a trained chieftain of the tribe. Now I am able to produce results which cause people to marvel over my healing power with the many medicinal plants found here in the forest of the Peruvian Amazon.

When the Chief's death left me depending entirely on my own knowledge, sometimes I had difficulties with my treatment of a sickness. When this happened I did nothing more than prepare with my own hands the extract of *ayahuasca* as I had been trained and then take it, various times if necessary, to find my error and follow the treatment exactly as indicated by the vine. This is why now I rarely fail to get the results desired. My patients have included the highest personages in the government. And the verifiable outcome of over fifty years dedicated to this work is ample testimony of its value and effectiveness.

If a person properly prepares and trains himself ahead of time, taking *ayahuasca* opens certain unused channels of the mind. The key *honi* or *ayahuasca* chants and songs that I learned actually initiate and channel the flow of visions. Later, as the scene progresses, it seems that half-learned, half-spontaneous chants sway the sequence and content of the internal vision message. My impression is that all this material flows from a preconscious level or perhaps even from some outside source. In the subsequent clarivoyant state, one's attention can be sharply focused and a participant can envision the interior functioning of his own body or, changing focus, can see within the body of a selected subject as I have already described. What one wants to see, near or far, appears; and if no voluntary direction is applied to determine the flow, the visions progress as in a kaleidoscope, or flowing one after another as the scenes in a cinema. The sense of time disappears and one becomes the master of the past and the future, also the sage of the plant and animal worlds. All kinds of life forms of the forest appear, usually followed by colored panoramic vistas and spontaneous music.

Ayahuasca can be prepared with varying ingredients and of different strengths, from a cold water infusion of the vine alone to a decoction boiled slowly several days in combination with the leaves of the shrub *chacruna* or *yagé*. The length of the soaking or boiling controls the strength of the potion. The stronger preparations should be drunk only by a *maestro ayahuasquero* who has had the kind of training I received from the Huni Kui, and even then only after the body has been conditioned by purges and a strict diet. A vigilant person should be present always to guide, protect, and watch over the session. This is essential, whether a person is taking it alone or in a group taking *ayahuasca* together. The most favorable time for seeing the *ayahuasca* visions falls at night, preferably in a setting of complete tranquility in the solitude of a camp deep in the forest where only the subtle sounds and smells of unruffled nature provide the background.

Through *ayahuasca* music—songs, chants, and whistled tunes—a subtle form of control develops; important elements of the vision progress and establish their own key melodies. Each natural object, be it animal, plant, stream or even rock, has its own melodic progression. By means of these sequences one can examine or enmesh himself within that object for a detailed examination of its nature and its properties.[1]

As Córdova paused my bewilderment must have been obvious as I tried to respond. "But Don Manuel, these experiences you describe have been so far removed from the life of our everyday world that it seems impossible to make it all credible to people without some special background for understanding such events."

So it appears, he replied. over the years I have come to realize that many people do not comprehend the interrelated elements of a healing syndrome that I have long since taken for granted. And regarding this, there is a word of caution which I must insist that you state specifically in anything you write about the plant substances I use. *It is very dangerous to put partial knowledge of potent jungle plant materials at the disposal of inexperienced and ignorant people.* I will give you an example. But first let me say that my cures of desperately ill people come from understanding the source of the illness, from a knowledge of which plants contain substances that will alleviate the problem, from adequate preparation of the plant extracts and proper dosage, plus—and this is very important—a careful observation of the patient's progress and modification of the treatment when necessary. My success is based on seven years of apprenticeship and over fifty years of experience. For people without adequate preparation and understanding to go ahead and study potent plant materials superficially and then experiment with them on human beings is an invitation to disaster.

At a small jungle town on the Rio Huallaga where I was making a collection of medicinal plants of the forest for Astoria, the company maintained a mahogany log-gathering station for the sawmill in Iquitos. When I was gathering some plants in the nearby forest—this was some years ago—one of the young men working on the log rafts came to me suffering from a very bad sore throat and head cold. I had known him well when he was a neighbor child playing with my boys in Iquitos. He approached me now, a well-built ruffian of a young man, to see if I could relieve his illness. With a bad cold he could not work in the water tying up logs into rafts.

Well, when I had worked with the Witoto Indians from the Rio Napo-Putumayo region I found they had developed an excellent remedy for this malady—the cold brought to them by the white man—and I was sure their remedy would help this young man. But I asked him to help me find the materials for his own cure, and this was a mistake.

We went looking for a certain tree inhabited by a special variety of stinging ant. When we found the tree I showed him how to capture the ants on a piece of cotton without suffering their painful sting. We put them one at a time into a bottle of *aguardiente* (raw liquor)—a dozen or so ants are enough. They carry a potent remedy in their stinger which is extracted by the liquor. I shook the bottle of liquor with the ants in it, and told him to take a tablespoonful every hour until he felt better, and after that to take a tablespoon every four hours for a couple more days. I also, without telling him why, cautioned him against drinking the liquor or consuming the remedy faster than I had prescribed. Now it just happens that this preparation, in addition to being a good cold cure, is a very strong aphrodisiac if taken in larger doses. I had prepared just enough to cure the cold completely if the remedy were taken as directed. Unfortunately I had to be gone in the forest collecting plants for several days, thus I could not watch over my patient. This would have made no difference if he had followed my directions.

The boss in charge of the log-buying station was a real ramrod, and a couple of days after I left he called the young raftsman into the office to see how he was coming along because his help was needed on the rafts to prepare a log tow for a tugboat that was in port waiting to go down river. This rough and raspy old Spaniard, whom I will not name, had been with the company a long time and was really past retirement age. My young patient reported that his cold was nearly cured, but that he could not yet go to work. His pants were bulging out in front from an erection of the penis that he could not make go down.

This aroused the curiosity of the boss who insisted, with threats of violence and dismissal, that the young man tell him just what had caused this interesting condition. Of course, the preparation of the remedy I had given came out when the young man told about drinking up the bottle of *aguardiente* at a much faster pace than I had prescribed.

The old man, who'd been a real *gallo* in his younger days on the river, should have known better, but he was now bored with declining libido and sexual prowess in his old age. He proceeded to prepare himself a bottle of liquor, ants added, and enjoy the effects. In addition, he told the tugboat captain, a friend of many years and about the same age and condition in life. Then the captain also took advantage of my cold remedy for its stimulating reaction.

Well, you might say that those two corrupted old farts literally screwed themselves into early graves, because that is exactly what happened. The original mistake, however, was mine in revealing to a patient how the remedy was prepared. Under duress he passed it along. But I no longer discuss my remedies openly or tell what they consist of and how they are made.

I have nothing against using aphrodisiacs for an impotent young man who wants to raise a family. In fact, I have helped several such people. But encouraging impotent old men in their senile, unfruitful pleasures inevitably forcing themselves toward an early grave is an activity which can hardly have my approval. Still, maybe there are worse ways to die.

15

Man of Medicine

Manuel Córdova, when he discussed with me the incidents of his youth, often revealed a surprising ambivalence toward his experience with the Huni Kui. On the one hand, he mourned it as an ordeal of trial and sacrifice, time lost. On the other hand, his every reference to the old chief Xumu was charged with the emotion of personal attachment, awe, and reverence. The training he received from this master in the forest was the single most important influence on the rest of his life.

From his own recounting of his adventures in a long and eventful life, it is apparent that only gradually did Córdova himself become aware of the scope of his knowledge and healing ability. Among the Huni Kui his life as their young shaman was curtailed in a stalemate between his tribesmen and their forest enemies with himself as prize. Confined to his village for safety, his life became unbearable and he took the first opportunity to escape.

However, as a result of his exacting and intense tutelage, Córdova took away valuable lore. He was given an incredible knowledge concerning the fragile functioning of the human body and its susceptibility to the potency of plant and animal substances drawn from the jungle. Córdova fulfilled a long-standing prophecy of the Amazon, and he served as the living link between two widely separated medicinal traditions.

A French missionary, Padre Constant Tastevin,[1] traveling on the upper Rio Tarauaca in the western Brazilian Amazon, spent time with the Huni Kui (whom he and others sometimes call the Caxinaua as well as Amahuaca) in the 1920's shortly after Córdova's escape from this area. Father Tastevin comments on the extraordinary knowledge of the medical properties of the forest flora possessed by these Indians. He says, "They know all the remedies of the forest. Every leaf, stem and vine they know and use as remedies: *dunu rau* against snakebite, *hui rau* against the sting of rayfish, *yuna rau* against fever, *uku rau* against cough, *buska isi ndau* against headache, *tchami rau* against venereal disease, *dete rau* against cuts, *tuku rau* against tumors, *kari sitsa rau* against skin ulcers, *imi rau* to limit human fertility," and so forth. Few other primitive people, according to Claude Lévi-Strauss,[2] have acquired as complete knowledge of the physical and chemical properties of their botanical environment as the South American Indians who utilize plant material skillfully, many times in multiply complicated procedures. This ethnoscientific lore has barely been tapped by the scientific West.

Dr. R. E. Schultes, Director of the Botanical Museum of Harvard University, a specialist on not only the botany of the Western Hemisphere but also Amazonian flora and particularly plants[3] with psychoactive properties, has remarked to me that "a major medical breakthrough is expected soon in the use of so-called hallucinogens to understand the workings of the human mind. And some of those so-called primitive medical practitioners of the Amazon region are a hundred years ahead of medical science in their knowledge and use of these substances."

Manuel Córdova's experiences foreshadow that breakthrough. Perhaps our troubled world could be transformed by a rediscovery of what these primitives already knew long ago. But adverse public reaction to the misuse of hallucinogens by both so-called seekers and Government researchers has led to a virtual cessation of new study and exploration. And the time is short, almost too short. Every day as the great avalanche of civilization encroaches further and grinds out of existence the last remaining nooks and crannies of the primitive world with their life forms and cultures, opportunities to retrace the adventure of Manuel Córdova diminish. Thus mankind walks a zigzag path through time, losing, it seems, as much as is gained. My own haste to share Córdova's experiences with others comes from a realization of what is about to be lost, and from my empathy with Don Manuel's frustration at having his healing accomplishments misunderstood and dismissed as either miracles or witchcraft. These superficial judgments give no credit to the intense training and long experience that, as Dr. Schultes says, put some of the 'primitive' medical practitioners of the Amazon hundreds of years ahead of medical science.

* * *

In February 1970 I went to Iquitos with a manuscript which became the book *Wizard of the Upper Amazon*, describing Manuel Córdova's experiences as a young man living as a captive with a tribe of forest-dwelling Indians. My purpose was to check every page of the story with Don Manuel for his approval; that meant translating from English to Spanish as I read. It took several days, as each of us had to fit the reading into our free time.

We worked at a desk in a large room just next to the reception area where Córdova received his patients when they came in for consultations. And he had to excuse himself many times during the days that we worked together in order to go out into the other room to see the people needing his attention. I used these interruptions to run through the coming pages and to get the rough translation in mind so that it would go rapidly when Don Manuel returned.

From those days the circumstances of only one of many interviews with patients remain in my mind. A young girl in her teens came in and Córdova went out to talk with her. I was only vaguely aware of the discussion going on outside, but enough to follow the changing mood. It began with the girl speaking in a very quiet and serious tone. The discussion went on and on, becoming more animated as it progressed and finally, rather suddenly, the girl broke out into laughter accompanied by low chuckles and comments from Don Manuel. The interview must have lasted half an hour or so.

When Córdova returned he must have sensed some feeling of irritation on my part, for he apologized for the long delay, saying, "*Mil disculpas por el atrazo, amigo, colaborador y compañero de la manigua* (A thousand pardons for the delay, friend, collaborator and jungle companion), but if I was going to help that frightened child, I had to gain her confidence in me and change her whole attitude toward her physical condition. You heard how she went away laughing—that was better than any medicine I could give her."

That incident sticks in my mind because it seems to symbolize Córdova's care for and empathy with his patients. In many of our discussions he has been critical of so-called modern medicine as he knows it from personal experience in Peru and from reading about it elsewhere. He says about the graduates of medical schools whom he knows as a result of personal observation and from correcting their mistakes, "*Estos doctores, todo cura nada sana* (Those doctors, a remedy for everything, a cure for nothing). Most of the doctors I know do not understand the real problems of their patients. They do not have the communicative skills nor take the time to find out how their patients really feel or how their condition developed. Another thing—they have no connection with the preparation of the medicines they prescribe and many times do not take the time to discover the patient's reaction. This lack of understanding and neglect of the healing process as it is taking place impedes their efforts to make people well and often results in malpractice. Such doctors often place on their patients an unnecessary burden of fear and anxiety. Medical schools should teach their students the importance of human communication and an understanding of the subtleties involved in what should be a warm personal relationship between doctor and patient.

"Recourse to surgery, though often unnecessary, has become the easy solution to medical problems the doctors do not understand or have not taken the time to solve. Surgical intervention should be used only as a last resort, but this is not how it is now—with the surgeon as the top man in the hospital. Why, the chief surgeon at the local government hospital is a former patient of mine. When he was a boy and had serious complications from a bad case of measles I made him well with an extract from the bark of the tree *ipururo.*[4] Recently he told me what he found on returning from leave—the young surgeons the medical schools are turning out now operate more like butchers than surgeons. He must have really read them the riot act after reviewing the cases treated while he was away."

To illustrate his comments on the medical profession, Don Manuel described for me several case histories of former patients.

One was the case of the chief of the criminal investigation section of the Iquitos police force who came to him and said he could not eat or sleep; he felt irritable all the time and could not even work. The doctors had X-rayed him and made all kinds of other tests on his body fluids and excretions. They had given him several medicines every one of which had made him feel worse.

"He told me," said Córdova, "'Now the doctors want to cut me open, but they can't decide where to cut.' After talking with him, I blended a mixture of the infusions of *icoja,*[5] *chuchuhuasha* and *bellaco caspi* tree barks. I asked him to observe and report to me on the results of this purge when he returned to see me the next day. I knew he was in for a surprise. My patient looked relieved and already much improved when he came back. With disbelief on his face he reported passing some four meters (about twelve feet) of the large segmented intestinal tapeworm called *solitaria.* No wonder he'd been feeling rotten! As a follow-up treatment I gave him medicine to eliminate any remaining intestinal inflammation and to strengthen his digestion. No need for surgery.

"I had another patient whose condition baffled the surgeons," Córdova told me. "One day a young boy who played with my sons came running in here asking for me in a big hurry. He told me the doctors told him that his mother was going to die if they didn't cut her open, and now she was asking for me. I went with him to see the woman, and on the way over, from our conversation, I decided she must have an intestinal blockage. The boy told me that his mother said she had not gone to the toilet for over two weeks.

"When we arrived at the house I found the woman in a semicomatose condition, half sitting, half reclining in a large chair. At first she would hardly respond to questions. But with patience and encouragement she became more responsive and finally she told me that two weeks before she had eaten a lot of *uvilla*[6] fruit, seeds and all. Well, *uvilla* seeds tend to stick together and those she had swallowed apparently had blocked her intestines. I talked with her until she was alert and relaxed and then told her I would bring some medicine that would clear the blockage. She thanked me—and I returned home.

"I had hardly gotten back home when the boy was there again, this time with a big smile on his face and a story that soon after I left his mother had gotten up to go to the toilet, but hadn't made it before the dam broke—and the house was a mess! He told me that he would come back and get me to see his mother again when the house was cleaned up.

"You can imagine what the result would have been if the doctors had cut that woman open. Just by talking to her and realizing the source of the problem, I had relaxed her enough to create a movement. Soon her condition returned to normal. That was several years ago and the woman is still well."

The inadequacies of professional medical services are of course not unique to Córdova's area of knowledge and experience. Kurt Reinhardt wrote in a paper for a seminar held at the Center for the Study of Democratic Institutions in 1969, "Medical *techne* in the Hippocratic sense . . . originally confined itself largely to prophylaxis and the techniques of protecting the integrity of the human organism to maintain or restore its stability and balance rather than venturing out into manipulating intervention and interference. [Now the] doctor-patient relationship is being sacrificed on the altars of social planning and programming."[7] With the trend toward cybernated diagnosis in conjuction with multi-purpose antibiotics, now microminiaturized, highly-sensitive equipment is put in place to detect, perhaps at a distance, significant changes in symptoms. The treatment is as precise and superficial as a computerized machine, and is the patient satisfied or made well? Richard Huelsenbeck,[8] once a practicing psychiatrist in New York, wrote in 1969: "I more and more hated the physician-businessman type who uses all the tests and all the tricks, but is not able to give the patient something substantial that gets him well."

The modern medical practitioner, in his impatience to avoid the patient's recital of multiple symptoms and get on with his sundry tests—blood count, sedimentation rate, electrocardiagram, etc.—may miss the very key that would unlock his patient's case, submerged somewhere in a perhaps rambling account of symptoms and medical history. He has more and more detailed information, but less and less actual texture and etiology.

Manuel Córdova, in contrast, has only his own acute sensory faculties available to him; yet he calmly looks at the whole patient and takes the reconstructed history of the entire body. By means of a set of astutely devised and subtly phrased series of medical questions or protocols, Córdova reconstructs with a patient the history of the problem, determining its nature, cause and location. Then, especially in cases of serious illness, he withdraws for a solitary night of analysis and contemplation of every facet involved. No longer requiring psychotropic stimulants, he achieves his penetrating analysis by spending the night in his hammock in a state of what he called *refleccion profundo* (deep meditation). According to his description of the process, he casts aside all awareness of external affairs and concentrates wholly on the problem of his patient. In this way he brings to bear the complete range of his memory and experience in diagnosing the cause and formulating a cure. He uses natural plant extracts that he himself prepares. Then he adjusts medication in accordance with the reaction of the patient to his treatment.

An interesting incident early in our association which drew my attention to Córdova's skill with suffering people occurred on our timber survey when we were together examining the forests of the Rio Nanay. In contrast to the turbid Rio Tigre, the Rio Nanay is a meandering blackwater river that flows into the Amazon just below Iquitos. We went up the Nanay by motor launch and one day stopped at the small village called Santa Maria de Nanay to obtain information from local sources. We had been tied up at the river bank not more than a few minutes when I heard a young woman's voice ask for Manuel Córdova. The pilot to whom she spoke said, "He is on board," and gave her a hand as she stepped up our steep narrow gangplank.

When she came around the cabin I noticed an expression of seeming adoration on her face as she greeted Don Manuel. After they exchanged a few pleasantries, she said, "Don Manuel, you don't remember me."

"I do," he replied, "but cannot quite recall the exact occasion of our last meeting. Forgive an old man his loss of memory."

"*Pues, por nada*, Don Manuel, it is for nothing," she said, "but I was on the point of death when I came to you a few years ago. You made me well when the doctors only took my money. I had given up hope and you made me want to live again."

'Ah yes, now I remember, but you must admit there is a difference in the way you look now! You came to me only the shadow of a living person, thin and pale as moonlight. Look at you now, plump and healthy! Follow my instructions and you will have a long healthy life."

"Don Manuel, I could never forget, and I am grateful to you for the health you have given me. May God protect and reward you. It is my great pleasure to see you again. Pardon the interruption, but when I heard you were here I had to come see you."

They shook hands and she turned to go with a radiant smile on her face. In a moment I heard her joking with the pilot as he helped her down our narrow gangplank.

When she was out of earshot, Don Manuel turned toward me and said, "You know, there are so many of these river people whom I have treated now that I can't possibly remember them all. It is the testimony of people like her that proves the lie of the grafting authorities who forced me into exile in Brazil. They could not do it now. When Cedron accused me of exploiting the people, I was in truth curing people the doctors of Iquitos could not help. How could I turn suffering people away from the door, people who had no other source of help?"

MANY OF THE PATIENTS WHO COME TO ME, ESPECIALLY THOSE OF MEANS are desperately ill and have been given up as incurable or dying by their doctors. When I cure them it is a miracle—at least many such patients and their families are fond of using the expression and the medical doctors seem unable to explain my cures in any other way. As a matter of fact, there is often no excuse for the patient's extreme illness. I will give you an example.

Alfredo, my youngest son, brought in a friend to see me one day. This young man told me his mother was having trouble with her legs and asked if I would examine her. They brought her to me in a wheel chair. Both of her lower legs were so bad from terrible inflammation and draining open sores that she could not walk.

She told me that several months earlier she had gone to Lima to visit relatives. While there, small sores had appeared on her legs and she went to one of the best clinics in Lima for treatment. The condition got worse rather than better. Finally in desperation the doctors had cut into her legs and even scraped the bone. When this did not help, they told her the only way to save her life was to amputate the legs above the knees. They said the condition would continue to get worse and finally would take her life. But she refused and said she would rather return home to Iquitos to die than have her legs cut off. When she got home her son suggested that she come to see me.

I told her that at least I could relieve the pain and could probably clear up the condition, which I diagnosed as erysipelas, if she would follow my instructions. I promised to bring medicine to her the following day, and they took her home, obviously suffering great pain. That night I prepared a special mixture of extracts from the barks of *chuchuhuasha* and *icoja* for her to drink as a blood purifier. Then I boiled in water the bark of the small fruited variety of the *taperiba*[9] tree to prepare a solution for bathing the legs.

After a few days of treatment large quantities of yellow fluid drained out of her legs and the inflamed condition began to clear up. Later, to restore the flesh and skin, I prepared a poultice of *sangre de grado,*[10] and in a few weeks this case of acute erysipelas was cured—a better solution than amputating her legs.

* * *

ANOTHER CASE BAFFLING THE SURGEONS WAS THAT OF A PROMINENT business man of Iquitos. While on a trip to New York he had a flare-up of stomach trouble that ended in his having a complete medical checkup in your country. He was told that he had a serious stomach ulcer. Immediately he returned to Peru for treatment. The Lima doctors wanted to operate, but they told the man's wife that because of his weak condition he might not survive the operation. So instead they came home to Iquitos, and one of my former patients suggested that I might have a better cure than an operation.

I instituted a regimen of diet, observation, and treatment. In three months recovery appeared complete. I used extracts of *chuchuhuasha* and *icoja*, and prohibited the drinking of ice water or other cold drinks. On the next trip the man made to New York, he went to the clinic for a checkup. They told him that the ulcer had healed, but that he should watch his diet and should avoid drinking all iced liquids.

Several years ago a former President of Peru was visiting in Iquitos on one of his political campaigns. He had suffered for many years from a stiff right leg caused by a knee injury during the early years of his military career. Someone told him about my healing record and the President called me in to see if I could help him. After he explained the circumstances of his lameness to me, I prepared a salve from a mixture of the fat extracted from the black boa, fat from a certain variety of *zorro*, opossum, and *babassu*[11] palm oil. This I gave to him with instructions on how to massage it into his knee. In a few days the lameness had almost completely disappeared. But shortly thereafter political tides changed and the President was forced to leave Peru, so I lost track of the case.

* * *

YOU HAVE ASKED ABOUT DIABETES. REMEMBER, AT MY RUBBER CAMP ON the upper Rio Tapiche I treated my own daughter for this malady? A longtime friend of mine in Astoria was the mahogany log inspector. He became a diabetic and this complicated his working life, because when he went upriver to inspect and measure logs it was difficult to stick to his strict diet and to take insulin shots when required. When he came to me and asked for my help he was in bad shape. He said the insulin shots were ineffective, the diet intolerable.

After carefully considering the medical history of his case, I gave him a purge made up of a mixture of hot-water extracts from the interior bark of the *tahuari negro*[12] tree, the bark of *chuchuhuasha*, and the bark of *bellaco caspi*[13], blended to fit the case. After the purge cleaned out his system I put him on a four-day diet of soft foods such as soups, roast chicken, and Quaker Oats. Then I prepared a hot-water extract from the bark of the small woody *ihuashtec* plant found growing among the rocks in the headwaters of mountain streams. I took the bark from the roots and lower stem of this plant and dried it in the shade. To make the extract of proper strength I then put ten grams of the dried bark in two liters of boiling water and left it for ten minutes, then removed the bark, and let the solution cool. In two weeks, while taking a teacup of this solution three times a day, my friend recovered from his diabetic symptoms. For his travels on the river I gave him a much more concentrated solution. He put several drops of this in his tea daily, and since then has led a normal life. That has been over fifteen years ago now, and when Astoria closed its sawmill and logging operations in Iquitos, he moved to Lima.

In another case a longtime friend of mine in Iquitos brought me the medical history of a relative in Lima with a severe, lingering case of diabetes that the Lima doctors could not seem to control. This time I sent the special purge of *tahuari, chuchuhuasha*, and *bellaco caspi*, with my friend along with instructions on how it should be administered and then followed with the *ihuashtec* extract. The sugar count went down from 486 points to a normal 280 in two weeks, and after three months of using my extract the diabetic condition did not return.

One day word came from the Hotel Turista here in Iquitos that the manager wanted to see me. When I arrived he introduced me to a well-dressed foreigner who turned out to be the Belgian Ambassador to Peru. Mr. Ambassador told me that he had met some of my friends at a military reception in Lima and they suggested that he come to Iquitos to see me. He then described at length a longstanding and intolerable case of lumbago that the best medical men in Europe had not been able to relieve. He told me all about the blood counts, X-rays, other tests, medication, and special diets, but he continued suffering. I told him that I would be back the next day.

That night I prepared a special blend of the extracts of *icoja, socoba*[14] and *chuchuhuasha*. The next day I took the bottle of medicine to the Ambassador at the hotel and instructed him to take four tablespoons of the preparation three times a day. Then I checked with him every day to see how he was feeling. The second day he already showed improvement and in six days seemed to be completely recovered. He then returned to Lima with a full bottle of my medicine to continue the treatment. In a few weeks I received a letter from him telling me how grateful he was for his restored health.

Several months later the Ambassador's male secretary came from Lima to Iquitos to see me, saying the Ambassador had sent him. The man explained that he could hardly urinate and that it was very painful when he did. He said the doctors in Lima wanted to operate on his prostate, but that the Ambassador insisted he consult with me before the operation. After going over the history of the case in detail, I told him that on the following day I would bring medicine for him to take. I then made up a bitter extract of three plants. The principal one was *yahuar panga* (blood leaf), from which I prepared an infusion made from the leaves with boiling water. When I gave this to the young man I told him to take three tablespoons of the extract every hour during the day, followed by a glass of soda water, and to urinate through a sieve which I gave him. In three days he passed two kidney stones covered with mucus and all his pain disappeared. After a few more days of medication he returned to Lima cured, no prostate operation needed.

* * *

On one occasion I returned to Iquitos from New York after many months' absence and one of the first things I did was to check to see how Manuel Córdova had fared while I was away. Arriving at his home late in the afternoon I found him conversing with an elderly man. We greeted each other warmly and after a few minutes Don Manuel excused himself and returned his attention to the visitor who had preceded me.

"How did your wife pass the night?" Don Manuel asked.

"The first good night's sleep in three or four months! I knew if I could get her here you would help her. But after returning home to Tarapoto from Lima she really did not want to travel any more. You cannot imagine the trouble I had convincing her to come to Iquitos to see you. But this morning she told me that she is glad she came."

After a few comments and instructions from Don Manuel, the man departed and left the two of us alone.

"What miraculous cure did you achieve this time?" I asked

him.

"Call it miraculous if you want," he replied with a twinkle of satisfaction in his eyes. "That man is an old friend from Tarapoto. His wife had a serious abdominal condition and went to a hospital in Lima for an operation. A serious infection developed and they gave her massive injections of antibiotics to control the infection. She recovered from the ordeal with an allergy to antibiotics that turned into an asthmatic condition the doctors could not relieve. When she arrived here day before yesterday my friend told me that she had not slept for over three months except for cat-naps taken sitting in a chair. She could not lie down without choking."

"How did you help her in so short a time?" I asked. Córdova not only answered my query but went on to talk of other cures as well.

THE SAME DAY SHE ARRIVED I STARTED WITH A PURGE TO CLEAR HER system of all the medicine they had given her. The next day, which was yesterday, I gave her my remedy for asthma, which will take about ten days for a complete cure.

I went to the market and purchased some *churos,*[15] those large forest snails that I have shown you. One of these I placed on a screen over a low charcoal fire until the juice started to run. This snail juice I poured off into a cup; then I added a bit of powdered balsa charcoal and the white of an egg. I gave her the mixture to take and it relieved her asthma enough to let her sleep lying down for the first time in three months.

You know, the synthetic antibiotics in commercial medicines and the synthetics in food in my opinion are the cause of serious medical problems. At least some of the cases that have been brought to me and called incurable cancer I believe have been caused by unwise use of these synthetic substances. The human body can eliminate natural substances used in medication, but when massive doses of synthetics are given as injections or by mouth they seem to stay in the body and become toxic. One of my main problems when a patient comes to me after lengthy medical or hospital treatment is to detoxify his system of synthetic medicines. Then I can begin therapy to overcome any malfunction of the body that may exist.

One day a young man came to the house and told me he wanted me to examine his father. I did not recognize him, and when he answered my question as to who his father was, I realized he was the chief surgeon of the local hospital. My further probing brought out the fact that the doctor had not been feeling well for many months. He had gone to Lima for clinical tests. When these were finished, the doctors at the clinic told this surgeon that he had incurable leukemia and that he had only a few months to live. They sent him home to Iquitos to be with his family. Now the son said that his father was moping around the house, just waiting to die, but the family felt something more could be done and that was his reason for coming to me.

I went with him to see the surgeon. We spent several hours together and talked about many things besides the sickness the man felt. It was true, what the son had told me, that his father was just waiting to die. At first it was difficult for me to get him to respond, but eventually his animation came back as he found that I understood his condition. Of course I could not talk to this man about removing evil spirits from his body. But we went into detail on the history of how his condition had started and the medication he had been taking. His skin was a pallid gray, his fingernails brown and the white of his eyes yellow—all indications of a toxic condition of the blood. I joked with him to change his mood and then I left, telling him that I would come the following day with medicine that would make him feel better. Just talking about his condition and explaining it to me, I could tell, made him feel a ray of hope.

That night at home I did not go to bed, but reclined in my hammock half asleep, going over the case bit by bit in my mind. By this time it was no longer necessary for me to take *ayahuasca* to see what was wrong with my patients' bodies. I could establish the connection by uninterrupted contemplation of the subject alone at night.

It was apparent to me that this man's problem was with the blood system and therefore I visualized the whole circulatory system. Nothing seemed wrong with the heart, the kidneys or the liver, but something seemed wrong where the blood circulated through the bones. And the plant *ihuashtec* appeared to me as the blood purifier to correct the situation.

The next day I made up a mild purge of *tahuari negro, chuchuhuasha,* and *sucoba* to detoxify my patient. I explained to him the effect and specified a bland diet. After observing the effect of the purge for two days, I started with the *ihuashtec* extract, instructing him to drink three cupfuls a day.

The purge started the change, eliminating the residues of the medicines this man had been taking, but a few days of the *ihuashtec* resulted in marked improvement. In two months this dying man was talking about going back to work, and in three months he did so, apparently completely recovered. I think his illness, from what he told me about its development, was complicated and aggravated by use of synthetic antibiotic drugs for various minor illnesses over a period of time. Leukemia is a disease I do not recognize since I do not analyze the blood. But the condition of imbalance in the blood system is something I can usually regulate with natural plant substances.

You ask me, is *ihuashtec* a cure for diabetes or leukemia? and truthfully I cannot answer. When patients come to me with the conditions that doctors by means of chemical laboratory tests have determined to be diabetes I can relieve the difficulty sometimes when professional doctors cannot.

My leukemia patient when he returned to Lima after his cure, went for a medical checkup at the clinic where his case had been diagnosed. The doctors there considered his recovery miraculous, unbelievable. And when he told them the circumstances of his cure they suggested that he very casually try to find out the constituents of the medication I had used in the treatment. Of course I saw through this scheme and bypassed his questions, revealing nothing to him. He finally confessed that his medical colleagues in Lima had asked him to try and discover the compostion of my cure. We both had a good laugh over the incident when I asked him if he told his patients just what was contained in prescriptions given them.

This reminds me of what happened a year or two after I returned from exile in Manaus. Word came up to Iquitos from Sr. Diniz in the Manaus office of Astoria Company saying that a local pharmaceutical company wanted several hundred pounds of the bark of the tree *pau d'arco* (called *tahuari negro* here in Peru). Mr. O'Neil asked me if I could furnish this material and I told him yes, that it was a bark I used. I was sure this request originated with my doctor friends Limirio da Sosa and Metrides de Lima because just before I left Manaus we had received some *pau d'arco* bark that came from the Rio Purus. They had started experimenting with it as a cure for internal tumors, *fibroma*. I heard later that the results had been only partially successful, and word came to me indirectly that they would be requesting from me a sample of the Peruvian variety of the tree. So the request was not a surprise.

I knew a small valley in San Martin where the tree was abundant in the forest, so I went there to cut and dry carefully in the shade nearly a ton of this bark. This was shipped to Astoria in Manaus and as usual I heard nothing more about it. However about a year later announcements began to appear in the Manaus newspapers which reached Iquitos, telling about the discovery of a wonderful elixir for the prevention and cure of cancer. And a few months later came an order for another shipment of *pau d'arco* bark. By this time I realized that my knowledge was being exploited without credit to the source. Under the circumstances I could find no more bark, and this resulted in an urgent but fruitless exchange of correspondence. Later I realized that the Brazilian Consul in Iquitos was without apparent reason cultivating my friendship. After a few weeks of this the question finally came up about the location or source of the *pau d'arco* bark I had sent to Manaus. I politely refused to divulge this information. This was not the first time other people have tried to exploit my knowledge of the medicinal properties of plants, and I was determined to stop it this time. But the story did not end with the Brazilian Consul.

Over a year later a lawyer from Cali, Colombia, came to Iquitos and asked for me. He told me that part of the tree bark I had sent to Manaus had been sent on to a pharmaceutical laboratory in Cali for testing. The lawyer told me that extracts had proven effective in curing cancer and more material was needed for testing. He said that the people in Manaus had referred him to me as the source, since they could furnish no more of the bark as effective as that which had originated with me. Of course, this lawyer wanted me to tell him where the bark came from or agree to furnish more. I politely put him off and he returned to Cali. Since then I have heard no more of the marvelous elixir, a cure for cancer, strangely discovered by men who were not able to furnish the raw material for its preparation.

Possibly they were right in saying that a cure for cancer had been discovered. The bark of *tahuari negro* I have been using for other medication. Who knows how many incipient cases of cancer I may have cured? However, there are two professionally diagnosed cases I can vouch for.

A boyhood friend of mine, now editor of one of the local newspapers, came to me one day and said that he wanted me to come see his wife. When I inquired why, he said the doctors told him she was dying of cancer of the uterus and that they could do nothing for her. He said to me, "She is suffering terribly and at least you can relieve her pain. You are my only hope and there will be no recriminations if you can't cure her—the doctors have already given her up."

I went to examine the woman and it is true she was not only suffering but in a terrible physical condition. I went home and prepared a solution from the bark of *tahuari negro* for a warm water vaginal douche, and another extract including also *sucoba* and *chuchuhuasha* to drink. In a few days improvement started, very slowly, but after several months of medication her recovery was complete.

More recently a neighbor from across the street came to me and asked that I come to her house to see the wife of the town shoemaker, a Señora Legia. I found out that recently she had undergone abdominal surgery at the local hospital. The surgeons found cancer of the upper uterus so far advanced that they just sewed the woman up and sent her home to die in a condition beyond the help of surgery. You can imagine the state of her health when I arrived to examine her a few days after the operation.

With an extract of *retama* flowers I reduced and calmed the abdominal inflammation in a few days and then started treatment with the extract I have already mentioned, made from the inner bark of *tahuari negro*. After about three months' treatment Señora Legia had completely recovered. I have also cured a number of cases of the benign form of this malady, before complications set in, the condition called *fibroma* by the doctors.

As with any doctor, however, my treatment of gravely ill patients is not always a complete success. For example two sons of a prominent Lima jurist, through a friend of mine in Lima, called me there for a medical consultation. When I arrived I found that their father, an old man and a very well-known retired Justice, was ill. Talking with the sons I found that the doctor had told them their father was dying of internal cancer. I went to see him with his sons, and then told them I would send medicine with instructions for its application. The old man was suffering great pain.

I knew that I could mitigate the suffering but was not sure the deteriorating internal organs could be restored at his age. From Iquitos, however, I sent preparations of *tahuari negro* and other plants. In a few weeks I received a letter from one of the sons, a professional doctor, saying that his father was no longer suffering, was animated and showed some hope of recovery. Later a request came for more medicine, and several months after that I received word that the judge had passed away quietly in his sleep. But his last few months had been without pain and suffering.

Occasionally, although it is seldom, patients come to me and I sense immediately that I cannot help them. When this happens I gently explain that I do not have the plant material needed for the treatment of their condition, and I suggest they go to the Public Health Service or to one of the many doctors in Iquitos. If they insist on having treatment after I receive the plants required, I am forced to give them a date beyond which I know they will not survive. You of course realize that even now I do not have the privilege of a licensed medical practitioner who is able to bury his mistakes without recrimination.

16

Shaman Master

Manuel Córdova was trained in and practiced a medicine essentially cut off from the entire Western scientific tradition. Although the esoteric aspects of that healing system are unique to the Amazonian lineage from which they came through him to the West, the basic therapeutic practices are familiar to us from the work of shamans, herbalists, and psychics throughout the world. The Western tradition *has* come to recognize the existence of a kind of energy medicine in which the remedy passes between doctor and patient (or initiated and initiate) as a pulsation, a telepathic wave, or vital potency contained beneath or within the materiality of the physical drug. The literature on this is extensive and includes biofeedback studies, parapsychology, experiments with psychedelics, concretization of the aura in Kirlian photography, and homoeopathic and other alternative medicines.[1] The reader would be best advised to examine my sources for more material on these systems.

Western doctors have been concerned with the observable chemical and physiological effects of drugs and surgery at the expense of other possible loci of healing. All modes of healing that restore health without fitting this model are considered miracle cures, which means flukes, coincidences, or misdiagnoses. Though we have dissected the human cadaver and the molecules of plants and minerals, we still do not know where the energy of life comes from, so we cannot know where the energy for healing comes from. The body has perhaps bioelectric, magnetic, vitalistic, psychic, and archetypal sources of power—fields which it would likely share with other natural substances. The path of healing can be through the vital properties of unpolluted jungle plants, the aura, the unconscious mind, or any other undiscovered channel. The personality of the trained healer, the initiated medicine man, is itself a dynamic element in the process. The word "psychosomatic," as commonly used, hardly scratches the surface when it comes to a healer like Córdova. "It is clear we are going out of the age of chemical and mechanical medicine," said William Tiller, Chairman of the Engineering Department at Stanford University, "and into the age of energetic . . . medicine." The Huni Kui, living in a rich spirit and plant world, never had any other choice. Apparently they chose, even on an unconscious level, to share their initiation with the West. Córdova became their last master.

* * *

Andrew Weil, M.D., in his book *The Natural Mind*, says "The essence of the (healing) process seems to be a kind of unconscious communication between healer and patient . . . through which the wholeness of a healer can be transmitted to a sick person."[2] Córdova himself marveled at the influence and force of his unusual mental powers. We were in animated conversation one day at his home with a group of the family including Doña Nieves, when Don Manuel said to me, "When the two of us are alone, I have an interesting experience with one of my patients that I want to tell you about."

A patient came in and he excused himself. Then Doña Nieves turned to me and said, "Mr. Lamb, in the past when Manuel required the stimulation of *ayahuasca* to divine the sickness and the remedy for a difficult case, I always sat and watched over him at night to protect him. Many times dozing there as he chanted to himself I have seen his visions also. It is an awesome and frightening thing just to experience a part of it. You wouldn't take that awful extract, would you, Mr. Lamb? Manuel doesn't take it anymore."

I explained to her my regret at never having had the opportunity to participate in a vision session with Don Manuel controlling the progression. But I assured her that I would not want to take *ayahuasca* without Don Manuel to watch over me and guide the process.

A look of admiration came into her face and she agreed, "Yes, taking it with Manuel would be the only safe way.''

In a few minutes Córdova came back, the crowd thinned out, and during a lull in the conversation he got up and motioned me to follow. We went out on Huallaga Street and down two blocks to the nearest beer parlor, where we sat down in a private room in the back. When the beer had come and we were alone, Córdova began his story.

MANY WOMEN COME TO ME WITH THEIR HUSBANDS, COMPLAINING OF difficulties with their reproductive organs. And I can take care of these problems. In the case I wanted to tell you about, a couple came to me and I remember a very strong impression that went through my mind as the symptoms were described to me. To myself I thought—what a beautiful, attractive young woman to be so afflicted, but I will cure her. When our discussions were done I told them that the medicine would be ready the following day. The plant extracts were picked up and I heard nothing more for several weeks. Then one day walking down the street I saw my patient standing in the doorway of her home. As I passed she spoke to me and asked me to come in. I inquired about her health and she replied that my treatment had eliminated the difficulty, with only one remaining problem. ''What is that?'' I asked her.

And she replied, ''Since I came to talk to you that day at your house with my husband, I have been unable to sleep at night without dreaming about you. And I want to ask you what this means.''

I replied, ''A doctor's relationship with his patients, to be effective, must be close but formal. If our encounter, resulting from your illness, caused you to have an undue emotional attachment to me personally it will now disappear. I am pleased to see you in such good health, and your dreams will not recur.'' She shook my hand and thanked me warmly for my help and I left. But I ask you, how could my mental impression of her beauty and attractiveness have registered on her mind, causing her to dream about me?

Another time an army captain came with his wife. We discussed at length the onset and persistence of a very painful irritation of the vagina. It seemed obvious to me from the response to my questions that no infection or organic condition was responsible. Finally

I asked the husband to return the next day for the remedy I would prepare. When he came, I gave him the medicine, but told him, "The real source of your wife's trouble is the unnatural positions you are forcing on her during sexual intercourse. If you really want her to recover, stop this."

"Oh!" he said, nearly jumping out of his skin, "How do you know?"

I replied, "Never mind how I know. That is unimportant. Just stop it for the sake of your wife's health. The remedy I have given you will help." Several months later the captain came and thanked me for the advice.

* * *

In addition to his perhaps novel but effective means of determining the basic causes for the dysfunction of the human organism, Córdova felt that his part in the healing process was not to eliminate or directly counteract the trouble, but rather to create a condition of harmony and stability that would allow the body to heal itself. His efforts seemed more to stimulate and direct the natural flow of healing energy within the human system than to combat disease directly.

Reporters have been notably unsuccessful in trying to capture the essence of Córdova's healing power in an interview. He said to me once, "These people smile and misunderstand what I am trying to say when I tell them that the operation of the human body is to me like a problem in mathematics. But essentially when you consider that the proper functioning of the body depends on the nervous system directed by the brain, the blood system controlled by the heart, and the digestive system supplied by the stomach, with all of these interrelated by means of various other glands and organs, mathematics is truly the only approach to adequate expression. It is a problem in mathematics even if I do not put numbers on paper to reach a solution."

These interconnected systems, to Córdova, operate like a series of simultaneous equations. Change a factor in one and the whole system is affected. And he said, "I cure people by knowing which part of the system is out of adjustment and then by giving that treatment which will bring the various interrelated systems of the body into harmony again. I have access to the brain with my words and to the rest of the body via the digestive system by means of natural plant substances taken by mouth or occasionally absorbed through the skin.

"Again I must repeat a warning," he insisted, "A partial understanding of my methods can be dangerous. Many of the plant substances from the Amazon flora are toxic and counter-effective if improperly used. Their application must be in accordance with the needs of the individual organism at the time of treatment.

"Many people, doctors included, don't understand my attitude toward healing. For example, recently a young woman with a very sick baby in her arms came to me with the card of a doctor at Clinica Marín. She said the doctor told her that he couldn't help her any more, but he thought I might. The child, two months old perhaps, was suffering from an intestinal upset—diarrhea, vomiting and fever—and had stopped nursing. The doctor at the clinic didn't understand the condition, the medicine he prescribed didn't help, and the baby was getting worse daily.

"I told the mother, whom I recognized as a vendor in the local vegetable market, to let me see her breasts. They were sour and unclean. I gave her a bitter-tasting purge to take right there while I watched, to be sure she drank it down. Then I told her to clean herself and the baby, to wash and change her clothes. I also instructed her on the food she should eat and why, and told her not to nurse the baby until the following day after the purge had taken effect. And I asked her to come see me then.

"In a few days they were both in good shape from my treatment. The last time this woman came by, she said that she had been to Clinica Marín to show her healthy baby to the doctor who had sent her to me. He asked how much I had charged her for the cure. When she told him 20 Soles ($1.00) he threw up his hands and said, 'I don't know how that old man keeps from starving to death!' What the doctor doesn't know is that I make people well more for personal satisfaction than for personal gain. Over-commercialization of the healing power I have learned to use could easily, in my opinion, result in the dissipation of its force."

* * *

There are some interesting parallels between research findings reflected by practice in the field of orthodox medicine and treatments used by Córdova. For instance, the plant extract of *ihuashtec* that Córdova found effective in controlling diabetes, he also used to cure at least one professionally-diagnosed case of leukemia, as has already been described in the previous chapter. Recent medical research has shown that raw plant derivatives have startling curative effects. In one particular case, medicine from the West Indian periwinkle, *Vinca rosea,*[3] reduced blood sugar in diabetes and was also highly effective in primary treatment for acute lymphatic leukemia.

In the past decade important new advances in cancer therapy have stemmed directly from new chemotherapeutic agents derived from previously exotic plant materials. Remember that Brazilian and Colombian investigators believed they had found something potent in the bark of *pau d'arco (tahuari negro)* obtained for them by Córdova, so potent they announced the discovery of an elixir for the prevention, treatment, and cure of cancer. Córdova's own account of using the extract of *tahuari negro* has already been related. Whether or not extracts from the bark of *pau d'arco* contain cytotoxic substances of importance to cancer therapy remains to be determined, but this tree is known to produce a complex organic chemical, lapachol.[4] A study of lapachol has led to the isolation of a large number of complex organic compounds, derivatives of hydroxynapthoquinone. Lapachol is found in the heartwood of *pau d'arco*; what its forerunners in the tree bark might be and what their pharmacological properties are remain uninvestigated.

It has long been recognized that cancer results from a condition of uncontrolled cell divison in the body, occuring when the normal mechanisms of cellular operations controlled by DNA and RNA break down. It is Córdova's belief that the epidemic condition diagnosed as cancer today is caused by excessive use of synthetic antibiotic substances, other synthetic medicines, and food additives. Andrew Weil, M.D., in his book *The Natural Mind*, has said, ''Penicillin, the first true antibiotic to be discovered, interferes with the cell-wall formation of certain bacteria, and bacterial cell walls are different in important ways from human cell walls. But many newer, more powerful antibiotics are toxic to basic cellular processes—processes we have in common with bacteria."[5] A recent biochemical hypothesis[6] suggests that synthetic food additives are absorbed through the intestines without being subjected to the digestive process, and thus do not—as natural food substances do—get re-incorporated into the body cells but instead accumulate in various organs where, over time, they can become toxic.

When Córdova proposes that complex natural plant substances have greater curative potential than do over-purified or synthesized substances foreign to the natural system, he is not without support in the field of science and the medical profession. Recent reports in the news media about both the failures and the dangers of uterine contraceptive devices and side effects of synthetic chemical birth control substances make us wonder whether some of the Amazon Indian tribes do not have safer and more effective birth control methods using natural plant substances from the jungle. There may be a whole undiscovered medicine in the rich and varied flora and fauna of the Amazon—a medicine sorely needed by a suffering and diseased planet, much of its people cut off from nature.

As the incredulous young reporter from the Lima periodical *Trinchera*, Roger Rumrill,[7] told his readers after he had spent some time with Don Manuel: "The writer feels like laughing over these comments that appear to be taking science by the hair. But there are the testimonial letters, and the 500 patients that Don Manuel treats a month. And there waiting in the hot nights of Iquitos, the grave faces needing help. . . . *Quien sabe si allí en las botellitas que entrega Don Manuel puede estar nadando un proximo milagro contra el cancer*—Who knows if in the little bottles given out by Don Manuel there may be swimming the next miracle against cancer." Who knows, indeed?

* * *

Generals, Admirals, Judges, an Ambassador, a former Peruvian President, and hundreds of simple river folk look to Manuel Córdova as the source of their health. Cultural differences, lack of understanding, the simple fact of the circumstances of Manuel

Córdova's life—these have impeded the extent to which his knowledge has been used. But recognition has still increased. PETROPERU, the petroleum company of the Peruvian Government, is in the forefront of the flurry of oil activity in the Amazon. When an epidemic of hepatitis occurred in their jungle exploration camps, the director of the operation in PETROPERU came to Córdova for assistance. His plant extracts proved effective in controlling the epidemic. Because of this, Córdova was offered the position of director of medical services for the oil company. He did not wish to accept this responsibility, but acts on a consulting basis whenever he is needed. Also, the oldest and one of the most highly respected universities in Latin America, the University of San Marcos in Lima, a few years ago offered him the position of Professor of Medical Botany. This post was not offered lightly nor capriciously, and Don Manuel did not turn it down without serious consideration.

Long years have passed since that young *cauchero*, Manuel Córdova, sat beside a jungle fire at night drinking *honi xuma (ayahuasca)* with old Chief Xumu of the Huni Kui Indians, learning to control the progress of his visions and tap sources of energy and knowledge beyond our present understanding. He least of all, under those strange circumstances, could have foreseen the path his life would take, with what sensitivity he would gradually, in some ways almost unconsciously, develop his powers for seeing the imbalances in an ill body and for knowing exactly what grass or shrub or tree would yield the cure. He developed a skill either lost by civilization or yet dormant in our species. Many men and women have credited him with being a most remarkable healer, a true creator of miracles. But Don Manuel realized that for all the insight he was an ordinary man leading a simple life. He did not risk losing his powers by inflating them, and he did not seek fame and wealth at the expense of the world he loved.

At daybreak each morning he went to the local river market to purchase the day's provisions for his household. On the several occasions when I have accompanied him, there was always a spirited exchange between him and the fish-vending women about the state of his cat's health. This perhaps mythical creature, because of her delicate and embarrassed condition, could eat only the freshest of fresh fish. The product available on any one day never seemed to be quite right. And the serious discussions I have heard about the condition of the cat in relation to the freshness of the fish have always left the market women choking with suppressed laughter.

One day Don Manuel and I had been sitting in the small open patio of his home, where a late afternoon breeze from the Amazon River stirred the leaves of Doña Nieves' many potted plants. Doña Nieves, sitting there with some sewing in her hands, broke into our conversation, "You know, I have often thought that Manuel should have a place in the country where he could grow and experiment with his plants, but he does not take my suggestion seriously. He just seems to want to live here quietly, looking after his patients in the daytime and, often, spending half the night back there in his laboratory preparing extracts for the next day."

"I bet he chants over them, too—back there alone in his lab," I commented.

"Of course," she replied with a smile.

And Don Manuel, chuckling, chimed in with, "What good do you think my remedies would be if I didn't sing to them? The Indians who taught me their secrets believed that words carried by the breath of their shaman had a creative power all their own."

Epilogue

Why in this age of scientific marvels, when both natural and unnatural substances can be synthesized, should there be any interest in the Amazon flora as a source of medicinal substances? I hope what has gone before provides at least a partial answer. In addition, some thoughtful people believe that the future of mankind on the planet Earth depends as much or more on our adaptation to the existing natural ecosystems found here than it does on future technological developments that modify the environment.

With the recent spectacular technological advances have come large scale deterioration and even destruction of important elements of our natural habitat. To avoid famine and pestilence on the Earth requires maintenance of world-wide energy balances. The collective vegetation, including the tropical forest ecosystems, provides a vital function in its capture and redistribution of energy from the sun. And we must work in harmony with this essential, living process, being careful not to destroy it. The use of knowledge such as that possessed by Manuel Córdova could be an important guide in figuring out how to accomplish this crucial purpose.

In his paper "The Future of Plants as Sources of New Biodynamic Compounds," R. E. Schultes comments, ". . . . the Plant Kingdom represents a virtually untapped reservoir of new chemical compounds, many extraordinarily biodynamic. . . . The flurry of phytochemical research engendered by the "Wonder Drugs" has barely scratched the surface of the Plant Kingdom . . . Less than 10 percent of the organic constituents of the Angiosperms (seeds in a closed ovary) are known, (or) fully 90 percent remains for discovery and investigation. . . . "

Rudolf Hansel, in "Medicinal Plants and Empirical Drug Research," reminds us that "The experience of folk medicine plays a large part in the discovery of active plant constituents, . . . frequently pointing out the type of pharmacological action which can be expected and later verified. . . . Pharmacochemical investigation of the Plant Kingdom is nowhere near its end."

The plant descriptions in the following MATERIA MEDICA include only those that Córdova, at the time he prepared this collection early in the 1950's, considered to have possibilities for commercial drug development. As a matter of fact his mentor in Astoria, José O'Neil, the general manager, warned him not to expose all of his medical secrets. There are many plants, not described here, that Córdova used in his regular medical practice, for instance, *ihuashtec* and *tahuari negro*.

Córdova himself expressed a certain sense of awe at his ability to heal. In terms of ordinary reality, the accepted frame of reference for our lives, there perhaps is no way of explaining his extraordinary accomplishments. The evolutionary process, stimulated by environmental change on the earth, has undoubtedly resulted in leaving many redundant or standby sub-systems in the information processing mode we call the mind or brain. Neurophysiologists agree that the visual cortex of the human brain, a recent product of evolution, suppresses the functions of many older parts of the brain. Nevertheless, these sub-systems still exist in the homeostasis of the organism, used by those who develop means of activating them. Perhaps wild plants, obscure jungle weeds and climbing vines, correspond on some deep level of DNA to the submerged messages in the chordate nervous system. Perhaps plants have a radical role to play not only in the origin of photosynthesis and the life chain but the unlocking of the hidden energies of the ganglia of higher life forms. There is reason to hope that these latent powers can be made accessible, especially for the purpose of creativity and psychic healing. Who knows from whence comes the only occasionally struck spark of human genius?

* * *

On a visit of mine to Iquitos late in 1973, Don Manuel made some remark about his life as a youth with the Indians. And Doña Nieves looked at him and said, "You are lucky they didn't tattoo your face the way some of those Inucuini and Capanahua did who used to come to our house at Tamishi Manchari. I still remember how their faces were marked up, and those tattoos stay on for life."

Don Manuel turned toward her, obviously recalling the young girl who had run away to live with him in a remote forest rubber camp. He reached out, tenderly placing his hand on her head, and replied, "Those Indians I lived with were too astute for that. They realized that I couldn't go trade *caucho* for guns with my face all tattooed. The traders would have known I was buying guns for Indians and would have stopped selling to me." At this Córdova held up his arms and looked at the bare inner forearms, one after the other. "They marked up my arms as a substitute for face tattoos. But I removed them later."

"How did you do that? I thought those marks were permanent," said Doña Nieves.

"If you know how it is put on, you can take it off," replied Córdova. "But on the face it probably would be too painful to remove tattoos. On the arms it hurt enough!"

On this trip I had come with a request from a Córdova patient in New York, who by word of mouth had learned that Don Manuel formulated a remedy for skin cancer. In this particular case, treatment years ago of a persistent fungus infection on the hands by X-ray had caused a deteriorating withering away and scaly condition that the leading dermatologists of New York could not halt.

A few weeks of treatment with a healing salve formulated by Córdova had initiated regrowth of normal flesh and eliminated the abnormal scaly condition. More salve was needed to continue the process of restoration.

When I asked Córdova about the jar of salve he had promised a few days previously, Doña Nieves spoke up. "What will all these people do for help when Manuel is gone? No one knows his secrets. And requests for help and healing come now even from New York."

Don Manuel, then 86 years old, drew on his pipe, expectorated loudly into the potted plants at his elbow, and, to fill the awkward break in the conversation caused by Doña Nieves' anguished question, launched again into the story of our encounter in the forest with Amazon swamp frogs that had learned to speak English. Again he imitated the night-call we had heard in the jungle, "All-right, yes; all-right, yes."

In the laughter which followed I realized that Don Manuel had given his answer to Doña Nieves' question in the mirth he had stimulated. Some questions in life are best understood when left unanswered.

Materia Medica

Those reading of how Manuel Córdova acquired from the Amazon forest his esoteric Indian medical knowledge and then proceeded to adapt its application to the needs of people outside the forest environment will perhaps also be interested in his more formal descriptions of some of the plants he used, along with an explanation of how he prepared the medicinal extracts that have produced spectacular healing results. Perhaps the presentation of this material will provide a point of departure for continuing research on the Amazon flora.

Following, then, is a translation of Córdova's report written originally in Spanish to accompany the plant collection which he assembled and sent to New York for identification and analysis in the interest of developing commercial uses for these medicinal plants. This material has been kept intact for presentation separately, in the form in which he wrote it, instead of being dispersed throughout the story. In this way I hope to preserve at least this small part of the direct healing legacy of Manuel Córdova.

The botanical names following each plant description do not come from taxonomic determination of the specific plants in Córdova's collection, since those plants were, as far as can be determined, farmed out to pharmaceutical firms for examination and thus were lost before scientific identification could be made. The botanical names come from crosschecking the local common names given by Córdova with published botanical literature. They must therefore be regarded as only tentative.

According to Ames, "When, unsupported by botanical evidence, we seek information about plants, it is apparent that common names in any language should be treated with circumspection and caution. All studies of plants, disassociated from a scientific nomenclature that is fortified with authentic specimens, are likely to lead to serious error and unfortunate misconceptions."[1]

* * *

Let me emphasize that these notes are not instructions for self-medication with plant substances. Mr. Córdova wrote these brief descriptions only for the information and guidance of investigators whom he expected would be working with the specimens forming his botanical collection. *To use these plant extracts without full knowledge and understanding of their effects can be dangerous.*

FBL

Manuel Córdova's Report

PROLOGUE

Medicinal plants found on the margins of the Rio Tapiche may render a great therapeutic contribution in the treatment of certain illnesses, as much tropical as those of other climates, depending on method of use, taking into account the symptoms and the requirements of the physician.

As a contribution to progress in medical and chemical science it is my pleasure to give some details about the properties and method of utilization of some species of medicinal plants existing in our Amazon region, that from my viewpoint have curative and antitoxic properties depending on how each is used.

In the thirty years of experience that I have in handling the diverse plants of this region, I have proved that these plants can be of great utility to medical science for immediate relief of many who suffer from illnesses that appear to be incurable. But in this I do not want to appear unmindful of the fact that Mother Nature possesses all, holding in her grasp the antidote for all the illnesses occuring on our globe. Even if it is true that in reality remedies have not yet been found for some illnesses that seem incurable, I nourish the hope that it will not be long until we discover the cure for Hansen's disease (leprosy), tuberculosis, and so on. Then chemical science can very well distinguish the quality of each one of these plants and indicate the proper therapeutic application of each, since on scientific study depends the success of each of these plants that I have applied many times with effects that have been surprising and results that proved satisfactory.

Manuel Córdova-Ríos

1. ABUTA

This vine is found in general in the uplands (highlands), among the palms called in our idiom *irapayales*, also growing in other locations but very scarce. It is abundant in the *caucho* type forests of the upper Rio Tapiche.

Preparation: This consists in making an infusion of 100 to 150 grams of this vine in five liters of water; let it boil for ten minutes, and leave to cool. When cool it can be taken by persons who suffer diabetes, without measured doses, i.e., taken as a substitute for drinking water in the quantity needed by the patient until cured. To begin this treatment, it is necessary first to have the stomach cleansed by means of a purge, alkaline in reaction. If after fifteen days of treatment it is shown that there is still glucose in the urine, then the treatment should be continued longer with a stronger infusion of *abuta*, made by using an additional quantity of fifty grams of vine in the same five liters of water.

Diet: The diet for diabetics: avoid greasy food, hot peppers, alcoholic beverages, and in general foods that tend to produce fermentation in the body.

Preparation (2): Make a maceration by placing 150 to 200 grams of the *abuta* vine in a liter of *aguardiente* (raw spirits) and leaving it for six days. At the end of this time it can be used as follows: for cases of women that suffer from menstrual disorders or inflammation of the ovaries, caused by chronic illness of the uterus.

Dose: A shot-glass full in a cup of coffee at breakfast time and on going to bed at night. This treatment should be followed methodically for fifteen days.

This same treatment with the maceration and the same dose can be used by women who for some reason cannot become pregnant. After this treatment is followed for three months it is very probable that fertility of the reproductive system will return. This same vine will serve as an aphrodisiac for impotent men, slowly increasing the level of energy and bringing back virility. In this case the method of preparation is to place 250 grams of *abuta* vine in a liter of *aguardiente* or other strong liquor, steeping it for fifteen days.

Effect: It has the effect of warming the blood and stimulating the nervous system.

Warning: It must be taken into account that there are varieties of this vine, but none is as effective as the genuine one that is found only in the uplands. In cases where the desired effects have not been produced, it is the result of using a similar plant. This is the reason why some people doubt the properties of this valuable plant.

Tentative Identification: *Chondodendron tomentosum, Abuta canducans* and *A. concolor.*

2. AZUCAR HUAYO or INCIENSO

This is a large tree with many limbs and abundant fine leaves. It grows only in the highlands and is very rarely found in the lowlands, much less along the streams. It is abundant in the region of the upper Rio Tapiche.

Preparation: Place 200 grams of the bark in five liters of water and boil for thirty minutes. Let this infusion cool and it is ready for use.

Use: This infusion is used for persons having rheumatic pains principally from lumbago, and kidney pains. Its action is diuretic and in general anti-rheumatic. It also acts directly on uric acid, to eliminate it.

Dose: Take a glass of this infusion three times a day before meals.

Tentative Identification: *Hymenaea palustris, H. courbaril.*

3. ACHUNI SACHA or REY DE LOS SANANGOS

This plant grows around the flanks of the uplands along the edges of small creeks. It is a small tree two or three meters tall. It is branchy with very long branches. The leaves are 15 centimeters long and three centimeters wide, and it has an abundance of light blue flowers that can be seen from a distance. Only the roots are used for curative purposes.

Preparation: Make a maceration by steeping the scraped bark of the roots in *aguardiente* and adding a cup of honey at once. Allow to sit for eight to fifteen days before use.

Properties: This is a stimulant for the body in general, principally the nervous system. It is used in cases of colds in older people, weakness, neurosis, and impotence in both sexes. The effects become evident about eight days after beginning treatment, when the patient begins to feel an animating reaction in general. When these symptoms begin, the individual should take cold baths in the morning to avoid violent stimulation of the nervous system and blood circulation.

Persons with rheumatism can also be treated with this medicine. For men who wish to increase their virility it is recommended that this preparation be used under medical prescription in accord with the age and physical condition of the individual to avoid the *unexpected* reactions.

Dose: Take a small glass or cup of this preparation in the morning and again in the evening.

Diet: Lard or greasy foods, hot peppers and highly seasoned foods should be avoided. The patient should eat roast fowl, eggs, fish, vegetables, etc.

Warning: This preparation should not be given to children.

Tentative Identification: *Tabernamontana poeppigi, T. sananho, Resedia* sp.? (Guttiferae).

4. AYAHUASCA

This vine is commonly called *ayahuasca negro* or king of the snakes. It exists isolated in the forest especially in the highlands. It grows with one main stem from which grow winding branches of considerable size and strength.

Preparation: Take five kilos of the vine, cut in short lengths and mash it by pounding with a stone. Divide in three equal parts and in a cooking kettle of twenty liters capacity place one-third in the bottom, spread out like a fan. On top of this place fifteen to twenty-five leaves from the shrub *yagé* or *chacruna*, also in a fan shape. Place another layer of the mashed vine and a layer of leaves and then the last layer of vine in the kettle. Add fifteen to twenty liters of water, and set the kettle over a slow fire to boil until about one-half the water has evaporated. The Master who supervises the preparation and taking of this medicine may take a full day or more to boil the liquid on a slow fire. When finished the liquid has a light green color and has the taste of water in which green corn has been boiled.

Method of Use: This plant extract is taken under the direction of a Master who produces it and selects the people who will take it under his care. He gives out the doses in a cup amounting to two or three mouthfuls as a maximum. If after a half hour no effect is felt, the same amount is taken again. It is important that to be successful this potion should be taken in a quiet place where interruptions and noise can be avoided. Seven o'clock p.m. is a good time to begin.

Effects: Lethargy overcomes the person taking *ayahuasca* and he falls into a half sleep. This is when the visions begin that seem more vivid than reality. One is affected by most agreeable auditory sensations, and the perceived visions put you into a state of ecstacy that you never want to abandon. The celestial fantasy is so sensational that there is no living person who would not find it desirable. Sometimes the whole vision is reversed and terrible, disagreeable impressions prevail. This usually happens when the person is not properly prepared beforehand with purges and special diets.

In the forest there are many tribes that take this preparation frequently—the Capanahua, Remo, Mayo, Amahuaca, etc. But they respect it very much, taking purges and dieting to avoid any disagreeable reactions.

Diet: The person who plans to take *ayahuasca* should go on a restricted diet for fifteen days. The diet should consist of dried or smoked unsalted meat, avoiding all sweets and greasy food. Cold baths should be taken every morning, and activities that produce strong body reactions should be avoided.

Use: The Indians take this potion to see things they desire, but conforming always to the truth; to prevent failure or to achieve victory in settling grudges between tribes; as a guide in the administering of some curative substance for sickness among them; also when wanting to discover some secret beyond their perception under conditions of their normal state of consciousness.

Varieties: there are many varieties of this vine, but the genuine effect comes from *ayahuasca negro*. There are unscrupulous individuals who do not know the various varieties and their qualities, but nevertheless participate in the popular diversion, or use *ayahuasca* simply to satisfy a desire for thrills that could be called *ayahuascamania*, i.e., producing side effects but lacking the benefits of real use. These people act greedily without realizing the profound secrets, available through the chants and songs, with people properly prepared and using plant extracts prepared by a Master *ayahuasquero*. Lack of confidence and unfavorable results come from giving improperly prepared extract to mistakenly credulous, ill-prepared people. In some cases it produces malaise, in others real illness.

This material, possibly to be considered a narcotic, can provide great assistance to medical science when and if it is tested by trained physicians or scientists, thus to give credit to its excellent effects and describe scrupulously the sorrowful songs that one hears in a state of trance—the reality of things revealed without a possibility of doubt.

Tentative Identification: *Banisteriopsis caapi, B. inebrians, B. rusbyana.*

5. CHACRUNA or YAGÉ

This is a small tree two or three meters tall. Only the leaves of this plant are used in preparing *ayahuasca*. These leaves have at the base three small spines or scales by which the plant is easily identified; it is generally found in low-lying lands. The *ayahuasca* Master often has these planted near his house. The leaves of *yagé* are placed in alternate layers with the mashed vine in the cooking pot to make *ayahuasca* extract.

These leaves, very well tested by the Indians, serve only as a part of the mixture, to make the visions clearer. Some tribes use various other leaves because there are localities where *yagé* is not found. These substitutes do not have the same effect.

Tentative Identification: *Psychotria viridis.*

6. AMPIHUASCA

From this vine a poisonous extract called *curare* is made. A forest tribe of Indians called the Tikuna prepare this extract to hunt birds and other forest animals that resist other, less potent, vegetable poisons. For this reason it also takes the name *ampi tikuna*. In their preparation the Tikuna mix a kind of hot pepper called *macusari* which has a high content of picric acid and gives it noxious power. The animals killed with this poison are safe to use as food. It has a violent effect on small animals, causing instant death. The Indians use it to hunt by means of a blowgun called *pucuna* or *cerbatana*, with small darts carrying the poison to the bloodstream of the prey.

Tentative Identification: *Strychnos* spp. and *Chododendron tomentosum*.

7. BELLACO CASPI or SUCOBA

This plant occurs in abundance in uplands as well as lowlands of the upper Amazon basin. It is a tree of medium size and height with few branches.

Preparation: Bark cut into short pieces or scraped fresh in the amount of one-half kilo is boiled in three liters of water until about one-half of the liquid has evaporated. When cool it is ready for use.

Use: This preparation is used for persons afflicted with colitis or intestinal afflictions. It acts directly on intestinal parasites, expelling them, and is thus a vermifuge.

Dose: Take a medium-size glass of this liquid at five o'clock in the morning on an empty stomach and then another an hour later, at six o'clock, followed by a glass of warm water.

Effects: This medicine will cause some discomfort in the stomach while it is active in the body, especially when treating an intestinal disorder. No food should be eaten until the effect is observed to be satisfactory. This should take place within six hours of the first dose.

Diet: Eat only bland food and drink hot tea instead of cold water. If the person eats, the effect of the medicine is nullified.

Other use: Women who suffer from leukorrhea (*flor blanca*) can be treated with this medicine effectively. It is necessary to observe a diet for fifteen days, eliminating all liquor, hot peppers, and grease from the food until it is shown that the milky mucous discharge has been totally eliminated. The patient should not take cold baths during the treatment.

Tentative Identification: *Plumeria tarapotensis, Himatanthus sucuuba*.

8. CURARINA or SUPAY CHACRA SACHA (CASPI)

This is a poisonous plant about three meters tall, reddish brown in color, wood very dense.

Occurence: Because of its poisonous nature other plants do not grow in close association with *curarina*. Nothing grows with it, no matter how high the surrounding forest.

Use: The original use comes from the Remo Indians (Inucuini) who have experimented with its application in cases of snakebite.

Preparation: Scrape the external part of the root and place the scrapings in 20 cc. of warm water and then strain out the bark quickly, and give the patient one swallow to drink. Apply the scraped bark to the area of the snakebite. After having done this the patient will feel within ten minutes that his life is safe and may continue work without interruption. This preparation is simple and is a proven strong antidote to snakebite of the most poisonous kind.

Therapeutic Application: Many times I have used the above preparation for toothache. Taking care in its application, you wet a small piece of cotton in the liquid and apply it directly to the tooth. The patient should take a cold bath and the pain will disappear. The leaves also have a therapeutic application for pain in the joints. In this case you soften the leaves over a flame and apply them to the area of the painful joints. This treatment is repeated until the pain disappears.

Many years ago when the production of *caucho* rubber was at its peak many people sought areas where this tree was abundant to set up *caucho* production camps. At that time I was a *mateiro* seeking production areas for the Borda Company, and a curious case came to my attention that alerted me to the profound observation of these Indians (Remos). When they saw that there was danger of their land being invaded by rubber cutters, they gathered this plant, *curarina*. Then they mashed up the bark, leaves and roots together in considerable quantity and in a woven basket placed it in the stream above the camps of invading rubber cutters. Within a few days the invaders would have to abandon their camp because, using the water saturated with *curarina*, there came a series of illnesses characterized by continuous fevers and swelling of the body. If use of this water continued, people died. I was aware of many cases of this kind of poisoning, which proves that this plant is very toxic if the extracts from it are taken in quantity or over a period of time. But in small doses it has curative properties.

Tentative Identification: *Duroia* sp., *Xylosma pilosa, Coussaria tenuiflora*.

9. CORDONCILLO or YANAMUCO

This plant is found in abandoned agricultural clearings in the uplands. It grows a meter or a little more in height, forming a single plant in the form of a reed, that breaks easily. It is about two centimeters in diameter.

Use: The original use comes from the Capanahua Indians who cultivate it as a protection for the teeth and to fortify the gums. These Indians give the leaves to their children to chew, telling them not to swallow the juice or leaves. Then they rub the teeth and gums with the chewed-up leaves. When this is done they rinse the mouth with water. In a few minutes the teeth start to turn dark blue and then become completely black. After about a month the teeth turn white again.

This treatment is done three times in one month and then repeated after a year or two. Then the teeth are good for a lifetime without decay or other disease. It can be used by a person of any age, but is most effective in preserving the teeth if started in childhood.

Tentative Identification: *Neea parviflora, N. floribunda*.

10. YANAMUCO BIJAO

This is a small plant of forest origin with potato-like tubers on the roots. It is abundant at the headwaters of creeks and on upland banks.

The Remos, who call this plant *minan*, utilize and cultivate it. The stem and tuber are used to protect the teeth. At the time of the new moon they chew the stem or tuber, off and on for three days, preferably in the morning, being careful not to swallow any. The teeth turn blue-black. They do this again at the new moon for three times and then the teeth are good for life. Rubber cutters have tried this treatment with good results.

Tentative Identification: *Neea* sp., *Capparis ovatifolia, Heliconia* sp. or *Calathea* sp.

11. COPAHIBA

This is a large tree with a long trunk and spreading crown. It is found throughout the Amazon, but two varieties are distinguishable—one from the highlands, the other in the lowlands. The first is the best, producing an oily brown sap that is of great value in herb medicine. The lowland variety produces a whitish oily sap with the same uses.

Therapeutic Application: The oil from this tree is used to cure blennorhagenous and external wounds of the skin such as burns and cuts. It is also used in cases of urethral inflammation of malignant origin.

In cases of blennorhagia and urethral inflammation, take a spoonful of this oil at five in the morning followed by a glass of tea sweetened with sugar, taking a cold bath right afterward. This treatment is repeated for three days, by which time the sickness should have disappeared.

Precautions: The person being treated internally with *copahiba* should abstain from sexual relations for fifteen days and should not eat greasy food, food seasoned with hot peppers, or drink liquor. The action of this medicine is purgative and diuretic.

Treatment for cuts: Put the oil on the part affected, after washing with warm salt water, repeating as necessary. After a few days healing will be noted, without danger of infection. In cases of older wounds, use warmed oil in the same way as above.

Tentative Identification: *Copaifera reticulata, C. officinalis.*

12. CACAHUILLO

This is a medium-sized tree with few branches, abundant on the banks of the upper Rio Tapiche and Rio Ucayali. It has abundant fruit pods during the fruiting time of this tree.

Preparation: Remove the hull from the fruit and then the soft covering from the individual seeds inside. Chop or grate the seeds and boil the pulp from five seeds with three spoonfuls of starch in a half liter of water until it reaches a colloidal consistency and takes on a purple color.

Therapeutic treatment: In cases of amoebic dysentery or intestinal parasites, take a glass three times a day before meals. In twenty-four hours, improvement will be noted.

There are many varieties of this tree.

Tentative Identification: *Theobroma subincana.*

13. COCHA TAMASHILLO

This is a climbing plant that grows on lowland creek banks near upland country. Its utilization comes from the Remo Indians, for cases of uterine hemorrhages or hemorrhaging from the mouth caused by some internal disorder. In cases of serious uterine hemorrhages in women, make the preparation by taking a quantity of this climber and making a roll with the stem and roots and leaves and boil it in three liters of water for ten minutes. When cool it is ready for use.

Treatment: Take a small glass of this infusion every hour and improvement will be noted right away with the stopping of hemorrhages, no matter how bad. After the third day of treatment the hemorrhages will not return. Sitz baths in the same infusion are also recommended, using a warm and more diluted solution, with six days between baths, just in case some vestige of the illness remains.

Tentative Identification: ?

14. CHIMIQUA or PAMA

A large tree found only in the highlands, occuring in groups. It does not grow along the streams. The fruit is edible, with an agreeable flavor, about the size of a grape.

Application: The bark as well as the resin has medicinal value. A maceration of the dry bark in liquor for eight or ten days can be used as an aphrodisiac for persons who have lost their virility. It is a diuretic and a disinfectant of the prostate at the same time. It increases bodily energy and can be used in cases of anemia also.

Aphrodisiac preparation: Place the bark in *aguardiente* or other strong liquor. It can be used to eliminate inflammation of the urethral canal also.

Preparation for anemia: Make an infusion with the bark and add sugar to make a syrup.

Use: Take a spoonful three times a day, before eating. The resin of this tree can be used as a plaster for painful muscles and dislocations, calming the pain quickly.

Tentative Identification: *Perebea chimicua.*

15. CHIRAPA SACHA

A medium-size tree usually found in overgrown agricultural clearings in the highlands not reached by floods. The bark, roots, and leaves are used with good results by forest-dwelling people.

Use of the leaves: In cases of erysipelas and swelling caused by it, put the leaves to boil, and when this liquid is cool enough, bathe the patient with the solution, repeating the treatment for three days, when the trouble will be gone.

Use of the roots: Boil the roots and leaves together, and apply this infusion when cool enough to wounds or sores that will soon heal. In cases of persistent skin ulcers, burn the bark, grind the resulting charcoal and apply this powder to the affected part. There is no skin ulcer that can resist this treatment.

Tentative Identification: *Vernonia scorpioides, Wulffia baccata, Psychotria calchlamps, Aegiphila filipes, A. peruviana.*

16. CHINTU or SACHAVACA HUASCA

This is a vine that is abundant in the upper Rio Tapiche. The principal root of this plant forms a tubercle about twenty-five centimeters underground usually weighing about five kilos.

Use: The Capanahua and Remo Indians use this plant for rickets, loss of strength, weakness and debility.

Preparation: Grate a slice of the tubercle into warm water and add a little fermented *yuca* beer (*masato*). This is then given to the patient to drink whenever he is thirsty. It acts as an emetic and causes vomiting, cleaning out the stomach without causing weakness. The treatment is repeated every eight days and soon the person begins to gain weight and strength.

In the case of alcoholic patients with bad liver, make the same preparation but without adding the fermented *yuca* beer. And give the same dose which causes vomiting. Repeat every eight days and soon the patient shows marked improvement and becomes normal. This treatment I have also used for cases of hepatic colic with good results.

Tentative Identification: *Clibadium* sp.

17. CHICURO PIRIPIRI

This is a small plant with small delicate leaves and on the root is a tubercle about two centimeters in diameter that looks like a small potato. The Remo Indians (Inucuini) use a preparation made from this tubercle as a narcotic to learn many strange things from nature. They scrape the tubercle into strong tobacco water, and the whole has a repugnant flavor. At the time of the new moon, in the evening beginning at dusk, they take this preparation and it causes them to vomit. At the same time they go into a trance. They pass through an enchanting sleep and take a cold bath very early the next morning and the effects of intoxication leave them.

Before taking this preparation it is necessary to follow a strict diet, avoiding greasy food, salt, sugar, hot peppers, and all liquor. The dose is repeated approximately three times a month starting at the new moon, and during all this time the participant dreams of marvelous, celestial things. Visions and fantasies appear in his imagination, together with real objects like unknown medicinal plants, the use of which is also learned along with the method of preparation and how the medicine is to be applied. Also in these dreams very strange songs and rare sounds are learned, called *icaros*, that are used later during curing treatments.

Depending on the constitution of the individual this diet and use of *chicuro piripiri* may be prolonged for as much as a year with the proper doses each month. During this period one learns so many things and gathers such special power that the Indian, the one who undergoes this treatment, becomes a Master, doctor, and sorcerer. They have great respect for one who can undergo this preparation because of his power to cure people of sickness.

The Remo Indians never part from this plant. Wherever they go they take it with them and plant it. To achieve a particular cure, first they sing and whistle the strange tunes learned during their dreams with *piripiri*. And it happens that if they abandon the proper diet during the time they are taking *chicuro piripiri* all these dreams they expect during the intoxication disappear as if by some magic.

Tentative Identification: ?

18. CHUCHUHUASHA HUASCA

This vine grows only in the highlands. The Remo Indians utilize the roots by scraping or grating into water and boiling the water until it is reduced by one-half. When cool, the liquid is used to wash skin sores or ulcers. Then they burn the bark and powder the charcoal and put this on the sore. This cauterizes it and in a short time it is healed.

Tentative Identification: ?

19. ESTORAQUE or SHIMIATI

This is a large tree that grows only in the uplands, and produces abundant fruit. When the fruit is ripe an oil can be extracted that has an exquisite fragrance, which is in the bark also. The use of this tree comes from the Capanahua Indians. They chop up the bark and put it in water and use this water as a bath to treat people with a bad cough or whooping cough. They also give this water to drink. It is very effective in reducing fatigue from coughing, stopping the coughing, and also in relieving bronchitis. As a precautionary measure, care should be taken with the fragrant oil from the bark and fruit. It irritates the skin, and must be handled carefully.

Tentative Identification: *Myroxylon balsamum*.

20. GUARIHUBA

A large tree of the upland forest, also called *coto caspi*.

Preparation: Chop the bark and make a hot-water infusion.

Use: Drink this preparation instead of water to avoid or relieve muscular pains. Body pains and rheumatic pains are quickly alleviated.

Tentative Identification: *Clarisia nitida*.

21. HUACAPURANA

A large tree of the lowlands, abundant in the forest of the lower Rio Tapiche. The bark is used as a maceration in *aguardiente* which becomes dark red. It is used to treat cases of anemia by taking a cupful three times a day. In a few days the patient will feel the whole body warming up. Continue treatment until recovery is complete.

I have observed many old people who are stooped and twisted and in pain. When they take the above preparation three times a day before meals they give up this life of pain in a few weeks, gain strength and can be useful and work again. A warning! It also acts as an aphrodisiac.

Tentative Identification: *Campsiandra laurifolia, Lacistema aggregatum*.

22. ISHPINGO or ASHANGO

This is a large tree that is abundant in the area drained by the Rio Tapiche.

Preparation: Chop up the fresh bark and put it in cold water for several hours. With this water bathe persons who have attacks of insanity or mental derangement. Also let the patient smell the fragrant oil extracted from the wood, and rub this oil on the temples and neck of the patient. Very quickly the patient will return to normal and be cured.

A maceration of the bark in *aguardiente* is also good for cases of nausea.

Use: Take a cup of this maceration twice a day alone or in coffee.

The distillers of *aguardiente* use this wood for vats to store their product because it gives a good flavor.

Tentative Identification: *Ocotea rubra* or *Nectandra elaiophora, N. reticulata*.

23. TANGARANA

A river-bank tree abundant on the Rio Tapiche and other rivers.

Use: During the period of flowering this tree produces abundant, brilliant flowers that are light pink at first, then turn red. Make a tea with these flowers to calm persistent cases of cough in children, especially whooping cough.

Also, boiling the bark with the flowers and with sugar makes a syrup to be taken once an hour for asthmatic bronchitis. This is also diuretic.

The tree is inhabited by fire ants. Gathering the flowers is difficult.

Tentative Identification: *Triplaris* spp.

24. YAHUAR PIRIPIRI

This small plant thirty centimeters tall is cultivated by the Capanahua and Remo Indians for its medicinal properties. On the root of the plant is a bulb resembling an onion. This is the part used for medical treatment.

Use: In cases of hemorrhages or bleeding from the mouth because of some internal disorder, take the bulb of this plant and grate it into warm water, strain and give the patient a cupful to drink once a day. In cases of hemorrhages from below give the patient a cupful of this infusion every three hours until the hemorrhaging stops. This treatment is accompanied by sitz baths at night.

In cases of dysentery the infusion of the bulb of this plant is also effective. The dose is a cupful three times a day.

For cuts, immediately scrape the bulb into a banana leaf and heat over a fire. Then place on the cut and wrap with a bandage. Leave until the following day, then wash with the infusion of the bulb. The wound will close and heal without infection.

Tentative Identification: *Dichromena amazonica*.

25. ICOJA

A medium-sized but tall tree, with a red-colored resin in the bark. The bark of this tree is used in many ways.

Preparation: Make a maceration by steeping the bark in *aguardiente* several days.

For rheumatism take a cup of this maceration three times a day. This will cause the body to feel warm and will indicate the good effect of the medicine. In a few days the pain of rheumatism will disappear. The patient should not eat greasy food.

This maceration is useful also in stopping hemorrhages in

women produced by arterial bleeding of the womb. Sitz baths are also recommended, using a hot-water infusion.

People suffering from jaundice can be cured with a cold-water infusion of this bark.

The maceration in *aguardiente* also acts as an aphrodisiac. For a fractured bone that has been set, heat up chopped fresh bark and apply to the limb at the point of fracture. This will accelerate the healing of the fractured bone.

Tentative Identification: *Swartzia amplifolia, Guatteria* sp., *Unonopsis floribunda.*

26. IPURURO

This small tree grows on the river banks usually with part of the trunk in the water.

Use: An infusion of the leaves is effective against intestinal colic. Takc a glass of the infusion and the intestinal pain will disappear in a few minutes. A maceration in *aguardiente* is a diuretic, also an aphrodisiac slow in effect. Many bars sell this preparation as a stimulant for the appetite.

For intestinal inflammation, chronic diarrhea with blood or pus, chop fresh bark of this plant, put it into water and strain. The liquid has an agreeable flavor of lemonade and can be taken as often as needed to stop the diarrhea and regain normal intestinal function.

With this medicinal plant I have saved the lives of many children during epidemics of measles when they have had no care.

Tentative Identification: *Salix martiana.*

27. MORURE

This large tree is abundant in the upland forest where *caucho* is found. Dr. Galdas of Brazil makes a medicine called Elixir de Morure from the bark of this tree as a treatment for syphilis. A syrup made from the bark is used for stomach irritations and intestinal disorders and perhaps even for ulcers, cleaning out catarrh and mucus and even acting as a cicatrical.

Use: Drink a small glass of the infusion made from the bark before meals for a month and the improvement will be notable. A maceration in *aguardiente* is a good remedy for malaria, being superior to *chuchuhuasha*. This drink is sold in many bars.

This tree can be confused with *tamamuri* and treatment with *tamamuri* will not give the same results.

Tentative Identification: *Brosimopsis obovata*.

28. MACOTE

This poisonous vine grows up into the trees of the forest extending from tree to tree. The flowers and fruits form at the branch nodes on the vine stem.

The Capanahua Indians of the upper Rio Tapiche use this vine to kill fish. They gather several bushels of the vine and chop it up. Then they choose a lake and scatter the chopped vine over the surface at night. The water turns black, and within twenty-four hours the effect of this poison brings everything living in the lake to the surface dead, including alligators, turtles, boas, etc. The Indians, from this abundance of dead animals, choose only what they prefer for food. The water of the lake stays dark for some time and is poisonous to drink.

Tentative Identification: *Serjania glabarata, S. fuscifola*.

29. MISHUR

This is a vine that is abundant in the forests of the Rio Tapiche. The Capanahua Indians use the curative properties of this plant to treat tumors and abscesses by scraping the bark and heating the scrapings to a temperature supportable by the body. Then they put the preparation on the tumor or abscess, repeating the treatment several times a day for several days. This will make the tumor or abscess disappear no matter how malignant. Sometimes the affected part turns hard but it can then be taken out or removed from the body.

Tentative Identification: ?

30. NIEVE SACHA

This plant, a meter or meter-and-a-half tall, is found only in the highlands and *caucho*-type forest. On the point of each leaf is a mark in the form of a cross.

Use: It is used for stomach trouble or intestinal irritations when the body will accept no other medicine.

Preparation: Scrape the root into warm water. Give the patient this preparation to drink until the stomach or intestinal pains have stopped. This should happen by the second treatment. In cases where the sickness is of long standing, the dose should be repeated until all signs of the trouble are gone.

Tentative Identification: ?

31. REQUIA or LATAPI

This is a large tree that grows in low, moist or swampy areas.

Use: As a medicine it is a strong vomitive-purge useful in cases of alcoholism and hepatitis, acting to reduce inflammation of the digestive system. It is also useful in treating anemia, malaria and beriberi.

Preparation: Scrape or chop the bark and put in cold water for twelve hours, then strain. Give the patient one or two cupfuls to drink and the effect will be noted at once. The medicine causes vomiting.

Effects: A few days after taking this medicine improvement will be noticeable, with greater animation and appetite shown by the patient. It is recommended to eat in moderation.

In cases of alcoholism the treatment causes all the excess of bile to be eliminated, regulates bile secretion, and reduces inflammation of the liver and spleen. With this treatment the desire to drink alcohol is lost for a considerable time.

In cases of beriberi the body should be purged with smaller doses than in the other cases. After the purge, make a sweat bath by boiling the bark and apply this to the legs. This will make the unnatural swelling go down.

Tentative Identification: *Guarea trichiliodes.*

32. RENACO

This plant (the strangler fig) starts out as a vine but forms a tree when full grown. It starts out growing on a palm or a tree and little by little envelops and kills the host plant. There are many varieties of *renaco* and the secret is to select the right one.

Use: In cases of pains in the chest and where the patient has coughed up blood because of lesions on the lungs, give a spoonful of soup made from the recently extracted resin of this plant on three successive days, followed each time with a glass of warm water. Then apply a plaster on the chest of the patient. In a short time the improvement will be noted by the elimination of chest pains. The patient should rest during this treatment. I have cured many persons with this medicine over the years, some of which were coughing up quantities of blood.

Tentative Identification: *Clusia insignis, C. spruceana, Ficus mathewsii.*

33. SANGRE DE GRADO

This tree grows around the flanks of the hills and near the headwaters of the small creeks flowing from the highlands. It occurs in groups. It is called by this name because the sap looks like blood. The sap is difficult to gather because it drips very slowly from cuts in the bark

Use: This resin is used to stop bleeding from cuts and hemorrhages and also for uterine illnesses. It acts to check bleeding. In the case of wounds and resulting hemorrhages, put the liquid sap of this tree on cotton or soft cloth and apply directly to the affected part, and leave until bleeding stops. In cases of uterine difficulties, dilute the sap in water and give it to the patient to drink; also place a plaster of this material in the uterine region.

The correct name is *sangre de drago*, but in local use it has been transposed.

Tentative Identification: *Pterocarpus draco, Croton salutaris.*

34. SOLIMAN SACHA

This tree grows in abandoned agricultural clearings made in the highland forest. It is abundant in the upper Rio Tapiche region.

Use: An infusion of the leaves is applied directly to the zone affected by an infection producing pus. Within six days it will be cured completely. During the treatment the patient will feel discouraged because of the pain, but this is only an indication that the medicine is working. When the pain is gone the patient will be well.

Tentative Identification: *Raynia speciosa, R. sagotiana.*

35. SHUCO

This is a vine making a tangle a meter and a half above the ground. On the root of this plant are found small tubers. The Capanahua Indians keep this plant hidden in a certain part of their gardens. They scrape the tuber into warm water and give two cupfuls to their young sons to drink at the time of the new moon three times a year. They give this to the boys from three to twelve years old. This treatment makes the boys grow strong and healthy, able to withstand any sickness.

Tentative Identification: *Vernonia* sp.

36. QUINA QUINA

This is a large tree of the highland in the forest where *caucho* is found. It is much used by *caucho* cutters to relieve pernicious and continuous fevers. It is similar to *chinchona* and its effects are the same, to stop fevers.

Preparation: Make an infusion of the bark which contains a latex. The infusion takes on the color of strong tea and is bitter to the taste.

Dose: Take a cup of the infusion three times a day.

Effects: It has a purgative effect. The fever goes down until it disappears, and the ill feeling is alleviated. In times past the *caucheros* made a maceration of the bark in *aguardiente* and used it, taking a shot twice a day as treatment and preventative for fevers.

Tentative Identification: *Myroxylum peruiferum, Capparis quina, Geissospermum excelsum, Zschokkea peruviana.*

37. TAMAMURI

This is a large forest tree with buttressed roots, found in both uplands and lowlands of the Rio Tapiche.

Use: This is a remedy for rheumatism.

Preparation: Make a cut in the bark and a latex-like substance appears. This latex is applied directly either hot or cold to the affected part, usually the joints. The improvement will begin to be felt in a few days. The rheumatic pain will disappear for a long time, sometimes not return at all.

The latex or resin is also mixed with *aguardiente* and taken early in the morning in doses of a small cupful. Sometimes it will cause a rise in body temperature. This indicates the good effects of the medicine, and the fever will go down after three days. The patient will then feel better, free of rheumatic pain. After fifteen days it is recommended that instead of drinking water the patient take an infusion made with the bark of *tamamuri* for another fifteen days.

Tentative Identification: *Ogcodeia tamamuri.*

38. VACA NAHUI

This is a climbing plant that is found in abundance in both the uplands and the lowlands of the Rio Tapiche and the small streams and also on the banks of the Amazon. The local people call it *curarina.*

This plant produces a seed that looks like a bull's or cow's eye, hence its name. The plant is also well known in Brazil. The fruits or seeds of this plant appear in abundance in January. The people that live along the rivers never go without having with them several of these seeds to be used in case of snakebite.

Preparation: Take several of these seeds and extract the nut from inside the shell, grate in warm water and drink a glassful if bitten by a poisonous snake. Also put warm gratings on the area of the bite, after making the bite bleed by an incision. Results will be noted very soon after application.

Tentative Identification: *Cissampelos pereira.*

39. AJOS QUIRU

This is a medium-sized tree found in abundance in the region of the upper Rio Tapiche. The forest animals when they eat the fruit of this tree have their entire bodies tinged with the odor of garlic, leaving the meat inedible.

Use: The Indians use this plant with good results to cure jaundice, indicated by the white of the eye turning yellow. It leaves the body of the patient smelling like garlic for some time.

Preparation: Chop up some fresh bark, making an infusion to drink which is given to the patient for three to five days each morning, followed by several cups of water and a cold bath. This preparation is also taken for muscle pains the same way. A heating up of the body is observed.

There are several plants with this same characteristic odor, in vines and small trees, that are used as maceration in *aguardiente* and infusion in water, but their effectiveness is weak in comparison with the tree.

Tentative Identification: *Gallizia corazema.*

40. ABUTILLA

This plant is a vine not more than one inch in diameter. It is rare in the *caucho*-type forest. Because of its scarcity in the forest the Remo and Capanahua Indians cultivate this vine for their needs.

Use: This vine is used by the Indians when a woman wants to avoid having children temporarily.

Preparation: Take three to five leaves depending on size (three large or five small) and boil them in a half liter of water until it is reduced to enough for a mouthful. This is taken every morning during the period of menstruation, and repeated during three menstrual periods—the same dose—with a cold bath just after taking the medicine. During treatment avoid sexual contact.

Tentative Identification: ?

41. ANANATI

This is a small tree, four meters (twelve feet) tall with a few small limbs at the top, and with leaves growing on the trunk. It grows in the upland forest.

Use: It is used as a vomitive purge and has the property of cleaning out all the impurities of the stomach and intestines, reducing inflammation and leaving the intestinal tract in a clean state.

Preparation: Chop the bark and put in cold or warm water and take out a glassful to drink. It is best to abstain from eating for at least six hours after taking this medicine, after which only light food should be eaten.

Tentative Identification: ?

42. ANGUILLA HUASCA

This vine is abundant in the forest of the upper Rio Tapiche. It has the characteristic of running along the ground. The thick stems hang from the trees. Branches sprout from the stems, and leaves are abundant.

Use: This plant is used for skin ulcers difficult to cure.

Preparation: Take the bark and dry it in the sun until it can be powdered. Apply this powder to the sore after it has been cleaned. It is very caustic and is used only in extreme cases.

Tentative Identification: ?

43. ANI HUASCA

This is a thin vine that has small leaves. It is found in humid locations around the base of hills in the uplands. It winds back on itself, forming impenetrable patches.

Use: It is applied to stop stomach and intestinal pains, and to relieve cases of colic.

Preparation: Chop fresh vine and boil it in water until an aroma of paragoric appears, then administer this liquid to a person with colic.

Tentative Identification: ?

44. CABALLO SANANGO

There are several species of this plant in the same family. They have different properties, but produce about the same effects. The above named plant is a small tree or shrub, used by the Remo Indians.

Use: It is used to treat persons who have been left weak by some sickness. It serves to strengthen the body.

Preparation: Use only the roots which are red. Scrape them into cold water and allow to sit overnight. Take a mouthful of this infusion. It will cause a slight dizziness and may also cause vomiting with general discomfort. It should be taken not more than twice in twenty-four hours. Take a cold bath in the mornings and avoid food cooked with salt, hot pepper, or grease.

The Capanahua Indians use a plant called *murco sanango* in the same way. This plant has a knotty trunk but the character and use are about the same.

Chuchuhuasha sanango, sanango de hoja azul, sanango huarmi, sanango amarillo and *murco huasca sanango* are all similar.

Tentative Identification: *Tabernaemontana* spp., *Rauwolfia duckei, Bonafousia sananho, Casearia* sp., *Anacampta* sp., *Rinorea* sp., *Faramea anisocalyx.*

45. CEBOLLA SACHA or AMANGAY

This is a small plant thirty centimeters tall with flat leaves that grows in the forest among the rotting tree trunks. On its roots is a tubercle the size of an onion. This plant is found in the forest of the upper Rio Tapiche.

Preparation: Boil several of these tubercles until they come apart, then strain and cool.

Use: This preparation can be taken in any dose during the day until the patient improves. It is used in cases of inflammation of the bronchial tubes and hoarseness. It is also used for asthma in more concentrated form and with a plaster made of the cooked tubers placed on the region of the thorax.

Tentative Identification: *Eucharis narcissiflora.*

46. CURARINA CHICA

This is a small plant one meter tall at most. It has no branches and the leaves all come out in a bunch at the top. These leaves are long and narrow. The trunk has rings around it at short intervals. The bark of the roots is light yellow with the consistency of starch.

Use: For poisonous snakebite and poisonous insect sting.

Preparation: Scrape several roots into water and boil until it turns dark brown.

Dose: In urgent cases give a mouthful of the liquid every hour; in less serious cases three times a day. It acts as a purge for the poison.

Tentative Identification: ?

47. CORDONCILLO NEGRO

This plant is three meters tall. The stem is thin and full of knots for a distance of some fifteen centimeters. It is abundant in the abandoned cultivations because the Indians cultivate it for its medical properties. The Indians use it against hemorrhages and against infection.

Use: For women who have just given birth, take an infusion of the leaves as a tea and continue three times a day; take a sitz bath on the same day of the birth. This plant is also used in cases of external hemorrhages as a consequence of a wound. But then the Indians use a species of small fungus that grows near the roots. There are only a few of these around any root collar.

The leaves of this plant show the marks of snakes' teeth in the form of perforations. It is not known what the leaves contribute to the snakes. But it is true that very early in the morning the snakes come and mark the leaves with their teeth.

Tentative Identification: *Piper* sp.

48. CADENA HUASCA

This is a climbing vine that clings to the largest trees of the upland forest. The male and female types occur separately, but their properties are the same. The female type forms a spiral and the male takes the form of a chain. This vine has a great volume of sweetish sap which flows as from a hose when the vine is cut.

Use: The watery sap of this vine is given to drink in cases of fever when the patient desires water. It is diuretic, making the patient urinate copiously, and it calms the fever in a short time. Recently extracted liquid also serves to calm bronchial irriations and facilitates breathing.

In Brazil this plant is much appreciated. The people prepare from its watery sap a syrup for cases of whooping cough, measles, and other children's diseases. They make the medicine by boiling the sap with sugar and call it Sirop de Muta-Muta.

Tentative Identification: ?

49. HUANCAHUI SACHA

This is a thin vine, not abundant, found in abandoned agricultural clearings of the Indians. The leaves of this vine have a nauseous smell. The Indians appreciate this plant for its effect that is opposite to that of *abutilla* in that it increases the fertility when women wish to have children after using *abutilla* to limit fertility.

Use: Chop up the vine and put in water. Administer this drink during the menstrual period on three following months. Take a mouthful of this preparation each morning beginning the first day of the menstrual period. This is according to the Remo Indians and has not been tested to check use and effect.

Tentative Identification: ?

50. RIHUI SACHA

This plant, some sixty centimeters tall with abundant small leaves, is an herb that grows in abundance in cultivated spots in the forest. Some people cultivate it to have in case of need.

Use: It is useful in case of an affliction called locally *rihui* which produces painful blisters around the waist which are very troublesome. In these cases chop the leaves and they produce a sticky juice which is applied to the affected region of the body. The pain stops immediately and with the third application the affliction is all gone.

Tentative Identification: ?

51. ITININGA

This is a vine that grows in the tops of the tall trees of the forest. It begins in the tree tops and sends its roots down to the ground.

Use: Once prepared this medicine can be applied for fevers caused by whatever sickness. High temperatures are lowered immediately.

Preparation: When this vine is cut it produces a juice which is mixed with water, half and half. This preparation can then be drunk for thirst, at the same time acting on the fever.

The Indians also use this preparation as a bath to lower excessive heat in the body; this way it lowers the temperature more slowly.

Tentative Identification: *Monstera falcifolia*.

52. ITININGA RENQUILLO

This is a small vine that grows on the understory trees three meters tall, putting out lots of branches at this level. It is abundant in the *caucho*-type forest.

Use: It is used to cure itch, mange and other skin infections.

Preparation: A reddish substance comes from the bark of this vine and that is the useful part of the plant. It is applied to the skin until the affliction has disappeared. This bark extract has the property of slowly burning and peeling the skin, leaving the new skin in perfect condition.

Tentative Identification: ?

53. SICHACHA

This is a vine that runs along the ground and from time to time sends up a trunk in the form of a small tree up to three meters tall. It is found mostly in abandoned upland clearings.

Use: The roots of this vine are used to give vigor to the skin of the head and help increase hair growth of those who because of some sickness have lost their hair.

Preparation: Scrape the roots and thus extract the juice that is watery and is used to wet the skin where hair should grow, as many times as necessary to obtain the desired results. A scientific study of the properties of this plant could lead to a remedy to eliminate baldness.

Tentative Identification: *Entada polyphylla.*

54. RETAMILLA

This is a small plant with many branches. The fruit produced in small capsules is a substitute for coffee, with the same taste and odor. It is abundant in the region.

Use: The root is used in cases of malaria and anemia.

Preparation: Chop the root and boil in water.

Dose: Once prepared, the liquid can be given to drink in place of water. It is bitter in taste. Its effect is purgative, sometimes causing vomiting, thus cleaning out the stomach and excess bile.

Tentative Identification: *Cassia leiophylla, C. fruticosa.*

55. MURCO HUASCA

This knotty vine sometimes climbs the trees or may be found running along the ground. It is abundant in the region.

Use: The Indians of this region use the vine to relieve a gouty rheumatism that is very painful in the joints and back. Also some fungi that grow on this vine are formidable against hemorrhages.

Preparation: For rheumatism make an infusion of the vine, chopping it into small pieces.

Dose: Take a glass full of this liquid three times a day for eight days.

In case of wounds or hemorrhages, scrape the bark and chop them, placing on the affected part.

Tentative Identification: *Maregravia williamsii.*

56. RENAQUITO

This plant grows on the top branches of tall trees.

Use: It is used to help cases of dislocations and fractures of bones.

Preparation: Make an infusion of the chopped leaves. In case of a dislocation, take the liquid and also apply a hot plaster of the plant material on the affected parts, changing it two or three times a day until the desired result is achieved. In cases of fractures, after setting, put a hot plaster of the chopped leaves on the place, where it has the affect of soothing the pain and assisting the bone in knitting.

Tentative Identification: *bromiliad.*

57. JOA HUASCA

This vine is abundant in the region of the Rio Tapiche. The name comes from the Capanahua Indians.

Use: It cures itching or smarting skin, no matter how persistent.

Preparation: Scrape the bark, chop and apply to the affected part of the skin.

Tentative Identification: ?

58. SHATANAPO

This small tree, two or three meters tall, is abundant in the uplands of the Rio Tapiche.

Use: It is used in cases of stomach or intestinal pain or inflammation.

Preparation: Scrape the bark of several roots and chop. Then make an infusion in water.

Dose: Take a small cupful three times a day before eating for three to five days until the pain is gone.

Tentative Identification: ?

59. LLAGA CASPI

This is a tree that I have found only along the Rio Tapiche and its tributaries. It is medium-sized, with few limbs.

Use: The resin of this plant is applied in treatment of skin ulcers that have been in evidence a long time without being cured by other treatments.

Treatment: Wash the ulcer and then apply the resin of *llaga caspi* to the affected part. If in five days there is no noticeable improvement, place pieces of the bark in water and boil until the solution takes on the color of strong tea. When it has cooled to a bearable temperature, wash the ulcer with this hot solution. With this treatment in a few days improvement should be apparent and a complete cure soon accomplished.

Tentative Identification: ?

60. NAHUI AMPI

This is a small tree about a meter tall. It grows in abundance on the highlands of the Rio Tapiche and is held in high regard by the Indians and others of this region.

Use: The leaves of this plant are used to treat irritated, inflamed eyes.

Preparation: Take several leaves and chop them up, mixing with a little cold water. Strain this liquid and immediately put drops in the afflicted eyes. Do this three times a day. Take a cold bath after this treatment. If no improvement appears in three days, repeat the same preparation and treatment but using warm water.

Tentative Identification: ?

61. MUCURA SILVESTRE

This plant grows scarcely two meters tall and is found in quantity in the highlands of the Rio Tapiche.

Use: This plant is held in high regard by the Remo Indians. They believe that it makes bad luck or sickness go away. It is used mostly on growing children.

Preparation: Chop the leaves and mix with cold water. Bathe children who are delicate in health with this solution every morning. The Remo repeat this treatment until improvement is noticeable.

The chopped leaves have a characteristic bad odor which causes these Indians to believe it chases sickness away.

Tentative Identification: *Petiveria alliacea.*

62. NAHUAYTA

This is a small tree with abundant branches found in the upland forest of the Rio Tapiche. The name comes from the Remo and Capanahua language.

Use: This plant is used to relieve rheumatic pains. Its action is against inflammation, and it is diuretic.

Preparation: The outside bark of the root is scraped onto a banana leaf, wrapped up and heated over a fire, and then applied to the painful area as often as necessary. In case of backache this preparation is applied front and back.

Tentative Identification: ?

63. MOTELO HUASCA or TAYA

This is a vine that runs along the ground and puts out small roots at certain places that have tubercles on them about two inches long. This plant is abundant in the Rio Tapiche region.

Use: Preparations from this plant are used by the Indians to protect the health of children at the age when they learn to walk.

Preparation: At the time of the new moon gather the leaves, chop them and mix with enough water to give the child a bath. Do this three times during the new moon. At the same time take the tubers from the roots of this plant and chop. This produces a milky juice. After each bath in an infusion of the leaves, give the child a rubdown in the milky juice from the root tubers. The Indians of the region believe that this treatment will make their children healthy, and that later they will not suffer from tropical sicknesses and can recover from any sickness that comes. It has been my observation that the true forest Indians seldom suffer from sickness.

Tentative Identification: *Lepidophyllum quadrangulave, Securidaca longifolia, Capparis urens.*

64. MARICA RENACO

This is a climbing vine of small size, so named by the Indians of the Rio Tapiche.

Use: It is used for muscular pains in the area of the kidneys and to counteract inflammation in this part of the body.

Preparation: Chop about a kilogram of fresh vine and make an infusion in the form of a tea. Allow to settle overnight. This preparation can then be used to drink in place of water, producing a diuretic effect, thus eliminating inflammation of the kidneys.

Tentative Identification: *Datura* sp.

65. MASHU SHILLO

This plant is a delicate vine that at short intervals puts out small leaves and at the same time forms tiny claws with which it climbs the trees (this all appears in the form of a flying bat). There are two varieties, male and female—the female with very small leaves, the male with larger leaves. On the root are small tubers. The Indians chop these together with the leaves, and with this mixture are able to make the wildest man tame or calm. Or the Indians use it to cure a person who, after a sickness, is left irritable or has changed character and is too passive. In this case they mix the plant extract with *chica (masato)* made from *yuca*.

Tentative Identification: *Pavonia leucantha.*

66. ESCAKERA HUASCA

This vine has the same characteristics as *cadena huasca* (muta-muta).

Use: The Indians use this vine in cases of asthmatic bronchitis, cough, and fevers caused by bronchitis.

Preparation: They chop the vine, put in water, and use it cooked or raw, drinking the preparation instead of water.

Tentative Identification: ?

67. PIRIPIRI IHUASHTEC

This plant is in the form of a reed-grass about a meter tall. At the termination of the stem small branches are put out and bear the flowers.

Use: The Capanahua Indians use this plant to relieve headache. Preparation: They chop up the roots and tie them on the head until the pain stops.

Tentative Identification: ?

68. INSIRA

This tree is five or six meters tall. It is found principally around lakes. Water usually covers the lower trunk. It puts out low branches. Its fruit is eaten by fish.

Use: The resin of this plant is used for toothache.

Preparation: The Indian, to relieve toothache, puts the resin on a small bit of cotton and places this on the painful tooth.The pain will stop and the tooth will be destroyed and fall to pieces in a very short time.

Tentative Identification: *Chlorophora* sp.

69. GAYO or TUMBO SILVESTRE

This is a well-known vine called *tumbo* the fruit of which is edible. The forest variety has a smaller fruit.

Use: The leaves of this vine are used by the Indians to limit the bearing of children.

Preparation: Make an infusion of the leaves in the form of a tea. This is given to the woman to drink on the third day after she has given birth; she then drinks a cupful each day for nine days. If she avoids conception by sexual contact for forty days after taking the treatment, this results in lasting sterility. The normal menstrual cycle is not interrupted but conception does not take place. About five months after this treatment the breasts stop producing milk and become smaller. I have used this plant remedy many times with the desired results and many years later the desired effect still remains.

Other uses: chop leaves and put in cold water. Add this water to beaten raw egg and take it to eliminate asthmatic attacks. Also the leaves wetted in *aguardiente* and tied to the forehead will relieve headache.

Tentative Identification: *Passiflora* spp.

70. YOCO

This vine is found in the highland forest of the Rio Napo. The stem is grayish green with white spots and reaches a diameter of three inches. It has many branches. The leaves grow in groups of four in the form of a hand. They are 20 centimeters long. The flower comes out from the branches and looks like a brush of the kind used to clean bottles. A fruit the size of an olive forms at the base of the flower and when ripe has three seeds inside. This vine when cut produces a yellow resin which will cause itching of the lips when a person tries to taste it.

Preparation: Scrape some 250 grams of the bark, put in cold water, and then strain. This will produce a liquid dark brown in color with an agreeable taste.

Use: The Secoya Indians drink a glass of this on the mornings they are going on a long journey or are expecting to do hard work. Thus they avoid fatigue.

Also they boil the scraped bark and take it in the form of a tea. This is a vomitive, regulating the bile. The Secoya Indians use it both ways and perhaps this is the reason they are healthy and strong.

Tentative Identification: *Paullinia yoco*.

71. ALLCU CHUCHO

This is a brittle, climbing plant that grows adhering to tree trunks from where it sends roots to the ground. It is not more than a centimeter in diameter. About ten centimeters apart on the stem are rings of nodes where the leaves and flowers form. The stem of the plant is scaly, light green, the leaves rough, five centimeters long. The flowers are bright red and white at the base where a kind of swelling forms, half open, where a sticky liquid gathers in small volume. The plant has a strong nauseating odor of dirty dogs from which comes its name.

Use: Indian women, when their breasts do not produce milk,

put the liquid of this flower on their breasts and after several mornings of this treatment increased milk flow begins.

Tentative Identification: *Urera lacinata*.

72. CHUCHUHUASHA

This is a medium-sized tree with many branches, abundant in lowlands subject to flooding (though the upland variety is more sought after). The tree is well known by the river people for its curative properties. The bark of the trunk and roots is used in several ways—in maceration with liquor, as a cold-water infusion, or boiled.

Preparation: The bark of the roots is preferred because it has a greater concentration of the curative substances. This bark is boiled in water until the liquid is reduced to a jelly-like consistency. At the same time separately boil a quantity of the leaves of this tree. Mix in equal proportion the liquid from the boiled leaves with the jelly from the bark. This solution is put aside until any sediment settles out; then the remainder is decanted off into bottles. The extract will have the consistency of paint that sticks to the side of the bottle when it is shaken, returning slowly to the liquid below.

Uses: In cases of leukorrhea (*flor blanca*) the woman should take each morning and again in the evening before going to bed a cup of coffee or tea or some other drink mixed with half a spoonful of the extract, continuing the treatment for several days until improvement is evident.

In cases of complications from giving birth take this same preparation. Also use vaginal irrigations prepared by mixing a spoonful of the extract of *chuchuhuasha* in a liter of boiled water. The irrigation should be done with warm water and should not be followed by a clear-water douche. This treatment is used each twenty-four hours at time of going to bed and is repeated until the curative effects are evident.

For skin ulcers put a spoonful of the extract in a half liter of boiled water and, while warm, wash the wound or sore. The solution should be 37°–40° C. to stimulate circulation of the blood and thus facilitate absorption of the medicine.

After this washing, lightly dry the wound with antiseptic cotton and then dust the area with powdered charcoal made of the tree bark. This charcoal is made by burning a piece of the tree bark. Then wrap the wound with a bandage. This treatment is repeated every twenty-four hours until the wound or ulcer is healed. As healing takes place the washings are spaced wider apart.

For a purge take the bark of the roots, scraping with a knife into small bits an amount of 200 grams. This is left to steep in water at room temperature overnight. In the morning strain this liquid and drink a water-glass full; repeat for three mornings consecutively. This acts as a purge and is used for persons who have suffered for a long time from a stomach disorder. It can be repeated every eight days when necessary.

Tentative Identification: *Heisteria pallida.*

73. CASHA UESHA

This is a grass-like plant that grows in abundance in the Amazon region. The white roots have the characteristic of producing at short intervals hard narrow joints that can be broken easily. The roots also have many nodes and extend out from the plant only a few centimeters below the surface of the soil.

Use: The roots of this plant are used principally as an aphrodisiac when a person suffers from lack of animation.

Preparation: Chop the roots and place them in *aguardiente* for ten to fifteen days.

Dose: Take a shot of this liquor as an apéritif before meals. This maceration has the property of stimulating the nervous system.

Tentative Identification: ?

74. NAHUI AMPI or YUQUILLA

This plant occurs in abundance in the region of the Rio Huallaga and the Amazon.

Use: The natives of these regions use the roots of this plant to prepare a remedy for conjunctivitis and also in cases of blennorrhea.

Method of use: For conjunctivitis, chop the roots that give a milky juice that is mixed with cold water. Then let drops of this liquid fall into the eyes twice a day: morning and night. In case improvement is not noted in two days the preparation and treatment should be repeated with warm water, as warm as the patient can stand.

Tentative Identification: ?

75. SHILLINTO

This climber is found on the banks of the Rio Huallaga and the other Amazon headwaters, and is known by the natives as a plant of the uplands.

Use: It is used to cure persistent sores that occur inside the nostrils. The use of this medicine is a delicate matter, and should be administered only by a Master or a person familiar with its effects.

Preparation: The stem and roots are chopped and boiled together in water to prepare a quantity of two or three mouthfuls.

Dose: Administered by a person with experience, the dose is three mouthfuls given to the patient at seven o'clock at night in a closed room. Afterwards the patient should lie down at once, protected from any drafts. He will note a rise in temperature that will become a fever lasting for three days. In cases where the fever has not shown up by the next morning, another dose is taken.

Diet: Eat nothing salty or sweet or greasy for three months, taking into account that after fifteen days the patient can eat food broiled or salted. All sexual contact must be avoided for six months. A special recommendation is to stay in bed quietly for fifteen days until the fever has completely disappeared.

Many people do not take the medicine of this plant because of the precautions required. Nevertheless it has the advantage of curing the most persistent sores of the nostrils.

Tentative Identification: ?

76. AJOS SACHA

This vine grows in the form of a forest and is abundant in the Rio Huallaga and Amazon region.

Use: It is used for colds, flu, muscle pain, and the beginning of rheumatism.

Preparation: Make an infusion of the roots of this plant that looks like tea.

Dose: At breakfast and lunch take a glass of this infusion.

Effects: The effects come slowly, heating up the blood and in a certain way giving tone to the bones. If some pain remains in the joints, take the leaves of this plant, warm them over a fire, and apply to the affected joint. In some areas the people prepare a maceration of the leaves in *aguardiente* and take this as a preventative against colds.

Tentative Identification: ?

77. ALGARROBO

This small tree, four or five meters tall, occurs only in the uplands of the Rio Huallaga. It is slender and very branchy.

Use: The natives put small pieces of the bark in *aguardiente* for ten or fifteen days and use it as an apéritif to prevent rheumatism, also as a slow aphrodisiac.

Tentative Identification: *Prosopis* sp., *Chloroleucon* sp.

78. INDANO

This is a tree abundant in the uplands of the Rio Huallaga.

Use: An extract of the bark, high in tannin, is used as a vaginal wash by women shortly after giving birth to avoid possible hemorrhages.

Tentative Identification: *Birsonia spicata.*

79. UESHA QUIRO

A tree abundant in the Rio Huallaga region. It is used in the same way as *indano* against hemorrhages. Also from the bark in combination with *indano* a useful and effective syrup is made by a person with experience. This syrup is used for women who have vaginal or uterine sores or ulcers, also to combat the affliction known as the yellow flux.

Dose: A shot glass full of this syrup is taken three times a day before meals for eight days.

Tentative Identification: ?

80. UBOS

This is a large branchy tree abundant in the Rio Huallaga and Amazon region, in the lowlands.

Use: A strong astringent can be made by boiling the bark in water, for washing wounds and for vaginal washes. For intestinal flu accompanied by diarrhea make an infusion of the bark and take a teacupful after meals.

The same bark burned to charcoal is ground and sifted and applied to skin sores after they have been washed in an infusion of the same bark.

Tentativc Identification: *Spondias dulcis.*

81. COCOBOLO or BOLA QUIRO

This is a medium-sized tree with few branches and dark, hard wood.

Use: The bark is used to make a maceration in *aguardiente* and is taken for anemia.

Dose: Take a shot glass full three times a day before meals as an apéritif. It tones the nerves and eliminates rheumatic pains. It is also useful to correct intestinal disorders.

Tentative Identification: *Schinopsis peruviana, Coccobolo peruviana.*

Literature Consulted in Plant Identification

Herrara, Fortunato, L., 1939. *Catalogo Alfabetico de los Nombres Vulgares y Cientificos de Plantas que Existen en el Peru.* Lima: Universidad Mayor de San Marcos.

Lao-Magin, Rafael. 1969. "Catalogo preliminar de las especies forestales del Peru," *Revista Forestal del Peru*, 3:2 (December).

Williams, Llewelyn. 1936. *Woods of North Eastern Peru.* Chicago: Field Museum. Botanical Series, Vol. 15.

Record, Samuel J., and Hess, Robert W., 1943. *Timbers of the New World.* New Haven: Yale University Press.

Anonymous. 1946. *Medicinal and Useful Plants in Brazil.* New York City: Brazilian Government Trade Bureau.

Bazan, Flavio, (no date, mimeo). *Lista Parcial de las Principales Especies Forestales Nativas del Peru.* Lima: Servicio Forestal de Peru.

Pinedo del Aguila, Victor M. 1967. *Evaluacion Economica de los Recursos Forestales de la Amazonia Peruana.* Lima: Universidad Nacional Mayor de San Marcos.

Seibert, R. J. 1944. "Forest trees and products of the Yurimaguas area," Enclosure to Memo No. 11, 331. U. S. Department of Agriculture. Agriculture Research Administration, Bureau of Plant Industry. Washington D.C.

Leahy, J. Gordon. 1945. "Brazilian medicinal trees and plants," *Brazil* (July), p. 14–15.

Sievers, A. F. and Higbee, E. C. 1942. *Medicinal Plants of Tropical and Subtropical Regions.* Washington, D.C.: Foreign Agricultural Report No. 6.

Chapter Notes

Foreword

1. Leary and Alpert failure: See Watts, Alan, 1973. *In My Own Way*. New York: Vintage, Random House. pp. 405–406–407. Also see Leary, Timothy. 1983. *Flash Backs*. Los Angeles: Tarcher.
2. Masters and Houston, whose book *Varieties of Psychedelic Experience* is a classic in the field of psychedelia, have gone into nondrug ways of inducing altered states of consciousness which Córdova has also done. See Avorn, Jerry, 1973. "The varieties of post-psychedelic expereince," *Intellectual Digest*, March, p. 16–18.

Chapter 1: Ayahuasca

1. **Caucho:** Dried latex from tree *Castiloa ulei*.
2. **Ayahuasca:** Extract from a forest vine *Banisteriopsis caapi, B. inebrians* or *B. rusbyana*, see Schultes, R. E. and Hofmann, A., 1973. *The Botany and Chemistry of Hallucinogens*. Springfield: Charles Thomas. See also Materia Medica No. 4, p. xxx.
3. **Honi:** Huni Kui Indian name for ayahuasca.
4. Huni Kui: Amazon Indians of the Panoan group.
5. Lamisto: Indian tribe of San Martín Province, Peru.

Chapter 2: Men of Chazuta

1. **Ampihuasca:** *Strychnos* spp. and *Chondodendron tomentosum*, see Vellard, J., 1955. "Les Curares," *Journal de la Société des Américanistes*. Paris, p. 73 and 77. And Laguna, José Villegas, 1952. "Estudio del Curare," *Anales de la Universidad Hispalense*, Sevilla. Vol. 13 (No. 1 and 2) p. 81 and 91. And Krukoff, B. A. and Moldenke, N. N., 1938. "Arrow-poisons," *Brittonia* (Nov.).

2. **Achuni sacha:** See Materia Medica No. 3, p. 175.

Chapter 3: Rio Tigre

1. **Leche caspi:** *Cuoma utilis*, produces milky latex used for chewing gum base.
2. Rosewood oil: Fragrant oil extracted from the wood of *Aniba duckeii*.
3. **Yagé** or **Chacruna:** A forest shrub, *Psychotria viridis* and possibly other species; see Schultes and Hofmann. *op. cit.* p. 194 and 195, see Materia Medica No. 5, p. 178.
4. Jívaro Indians: Amazon tribe from Ecuador-Peru border area, see Harner, Michael, 1972. *The Jívaro*. Garden City: Doubleday/Natural History Press.
5. Murato Indians: Amazon tribe from the Rio Pastaza area of Peru.
6. Nauta: Marañon River town below the mouth of the Rio Tigre.
7. **Cedar:** Spanish cedar, *Cedrela* spp.
8. **Mahogany:** *Swietenia macrophylla*, called *águano* in Peru.
9. **Aguanilla:** *Virola* sp.
10. **Pashaco:** *Acacia paniculata* and *A*. spp.
11. **Catáhua:** *Hura crepitans* with caustic latex in bark.
12. **Supai chacra caspi:** See Materia Medica No. 8, p. 180.

Chapter 4: Winged Death

1. Inucuini: Tribe or clan of the Panoan group also called Remo, see de Carvalho, Braulino, 1931. "Commissao de Limites Brasil-Peru" (1928). *Boletin de Museu Nacional: Antropologia*. Rio de Janeiro. Vol. 7, p. 255–256; and Oppenheim, Victor. 1971. *Explorers Journal*. Vol. 49, p. 167; and *Handbook of the South American Indians*, Bureau of American Ethnology, Smithsonian Institute, Bulletin No. 143.
2. Dunduri: Log drum, see Izaguirre, Padre Fray Bernardino. 1922 Historia de los Misiones Franciscanas y narracion de los progresos de la geografia en el oriente del Peru. Lima. Vol. 25, p. 435; and Oppenheim, Victor, 1971. "Under the Southern Cross," *Explorers Journal*, Vol. 49, p. 167; and Oppenheim, V., 1936. "Notas Ethnographicas sobre os Indigenas do Alto

Juruá e Valle do Ucayali,'' *Annaes da Academia Brasileira de Sciencias*, Vol. 8, p. 152.

3. Jungle Fever: See Izaguirre, *op. cit.* Padre Enríque cured of fever by Remo Indians in addition to Córdova's story is recounted in Vol. 25, p. 249.

Chapter 5: Poisoned Rio Javarí

1. Villarejo, Avencio. 1952. *Asi Es La Selva*. 2d ed. Lima, Peru.
2. **Supai Chacra Caspi:** See Materia Medica No. 8, p. 180.
3. Leoncito: *Cebuella pygmaea*.
4. **Balata:** A latex-like gum produced from the bark of the Masaranduba tree, *Manilkara huberi*.
5. In the late 1960's the Padres of the Maryknoll Mission and workers from the Summer Institute of Linguistics with a base of operations at Yarinacocha near Pucallpa have both tried to make contact with the trouble makers of the Rio Blanco area without success.

Chapter 6: The Capanahua

1. Pedernal Stone: Perhaps containing lithium.
2. **Achiote:** *Bixa orellana*.
3. **Huito:** *Jenipe americana*.
4. **Huangana:** *Dicotyles labiatus*.
5. **Chicuro-piripiri:** See Materia Medica No. 17, p. 185.
6. Harvey Bassler: Geological field exploration during the 1920's in the Peruvian Amazon region is described by Edson, Lee. 1982. ''The Collector.'' *The Lamp* (Exxon shareholders journal) 64(4):13–15.
7. Yacumama: Edson (*op. cit.*) mentions that the Bassler amphibian and reptile collections are now at the American Museum of Natural History of New York. Therefore the vertebrae and scales from the skin of the large boa taken at the petroleum exploration camp mentioned by Córdova should be in the Bassler collection at the Museum in New York. Also Perry, Richard. 1970. *The World of the Jaguar*. New York: Taplinger, pp. 74–100 gives an excellent review of the literature on the large boas.
8. Xanada: Indian village where Córdova lived with the Huni Kui.

See *Wizard of the Upper Amazon.*

9. Rio de las Piedras: Tributary of the Rio Madre de Dios.
10. **Ihuashtec:** An unidentified woody plant growing among the rocks in the small streams of the uplands, and sometimes during high water covered with water. The woody roots of this plant extend for long distances among the rocks and it is from these roots that the medicinal bark is taken.
11. Requena Convent: See Izaguirre *op. cit.*

Chapter 7: Life at Águano Isla

1. Restinga: Brazilian word for bank or ridge.
2. **Huacapu:** *Voucapuoa americana.*
3. **Shapaja:** *Atalea speciosa.*
4. **Pona:** *Socrates durissima* (= *Iriartea exorrhiza*).
5. Lunar cycle: See Beeson, C. F. 1946. "Forestry, horticulture and the moon." *Forestry Abstracts* 8(2):191–97. And "The moon and plant growth." *Nature* (London). 158:572–73. (1946).
6. **Charapas:** *Podocnemis sextuburculata.*
7. **Taracayas:** *Podocnemis expansa.*

Chapter 8: Fighting Cocks

1. **Retama:** *Cassia loretensis, C. marginata.*
2. **Retamilla:** See Materia Medica No. 54, p. 200.
3. **Chuchuhuasha:** See Materia Medica No. 72, p. 207.

Chapter 9: Exile and Return

1. **Tahuari negro:** *Tabebuia* sp.
2. **Pau d'arco:** *Tabebuia* sp.
3. Report: Materia Medica, p. 173.
4. **Oje:** *Ficus glabarata, F. anthelmintica.*
5. **Barbasco:** *Lonchocarpus utilis*, rotenone extracted from the roots.

Chapter 10: Curare from Rio Sisa

1. Pedernal Stone: See Notes, Chapter 6.

Chapter 11: Arab Surgery

Chapter 12: Rio Napo

1. **Yoco:** *Paulinia yoco*, see Schultes, R. E. 1942. "Yoco: A Stimulant of Southern Columbia." *Botanical Museum Leaflet*. Harvard University, Vol. 10, No. 10, pp. 301–324.
2. Uta: Leishmaniasis, infection of the blood with flagellate protozoans. See Kelly, Brian and London, Mark. 1983. *Amazon*. New York: Harcourt, Brace, Jovanovich, pp. 232–239.
3. **Rumosarsa:** *Smilax* sp./ Sarsaparilla: *Smilax officinalis*.
4. **Macote:** See Materia Medica No. 28, p. 190.
5. **Oje:** *Ficus glabarata, F. anthelmintica*.

Chapter 13: El Botanico

1. **Sanango:** See Materia Medica No. 44, p. 196.
2. Report: See Materia Medica.
3. Revista Trinchera Peruana. Ano. II No. 6, Junio-Julio. 1971.
4. **Abutilla:** See Materia Medica No. 40, p. 195.
5. **Gayo** or **tumbo:** See Materia Medica No. 69, p.205.
6. Scientific method: Bross, I. D. J. 1972. "Scientific strategies in human affairs: use of deep mathematical models." *Transactions of N. Y. Acad. of Sciences*. Ser. II, Vol. 34, No. 3 p. 187. "If scientists are to play a more constructive role in resolving the major problems of our society, there will have to be some drastic modifications in the prevailing scientific strategies, tactics and operating procedures."
7. Janeway, Elizabeth, 1973. "Beyond Stonehenge," Book review. *New York Times Book Review Section*. July 29, 1973. p. 17.
8. This commentary is found in De Mille, Richard. Editor. 1984. *The Don Juan Papers: Further Castaneda Controversies*. Santa Barbara: Ross-Erikson. pp. 94–98.
9. As a collaborator of his for more than 15 years, I have given my opinion on this subject in the following publications: Lamb, F. Bruce. 1981. "Wizard of the Upper Amazon as Ethnography." *Current Anthropology* 22(5):577–580. And 1981. "Comment on Boch's Review of the *Don Juan Papers*." *American Anthropologist* 83(3):641. And 1984. "Wizard of the Upper Amazon: Authentic or Fake Ethnology." in *Authentizität In Den Sozialwissenschaften*. Edited by Hans Peter Duerr. Frankfurt: Surkamp. In Press.

Chapter 14: Uncanny Knowledge

1. Manuel Córdova took *ayahuasca* extract himself in order to find out the nature of his patient's illness and to determine an effective treatment. He did not give *ayahuasca* to his patients as part of the treatment. Others report healers taking *ayahuasca* with their patients as part of the healing process. See Weil, Andrew. 1983. *Health and Healing*. Boston: Houghton Mifflin. pp. 158–160. And Dobkin de Rios, Marlene. 1972. *Visionary Vine*. Prospect Heights (Ill.): Waveland Press. pp. 99–116. And 1984. *Hallucinogens: Cross-Cultural Perspective*. Albuquerque: University of New Mexico Press. pp. 185–189.

Chapter 15: Man of Medicine

1. Tastevin, Constant, 1926. "Le Haut Tarauaca," *La Géographie*: Terre-Air-Mer Vol. 45, pp. 159-175.
2. Lévi-Strauss, Claude, 1948. "The Use of Wild Plants in Tropical South America," in *Handbook of South American Indians*. Vol. 6, p. 484. Bureau of Ethnology, Smithsonian Institute, Bulletin 143.
3. Psychoactive plants: See Schultes, R. E. and Hofmann, A., 1973. *The Botany and Chemistry of Hallucinogens. op. cit.*
4. **Ipururo:** *Salix martiana*, see Materia Medica, No. 26, p. 189.
5. **Chuchuhuasha** and **icoja:** See Materia Medica, No. 72, p. 207 & No. 25, p. 188.
6. **Uvilla:** *Eugenia uvaia.*
7. Reinhardt, Kurt, 1969. "Medical Ethics," *The Center Magazine*. Vol. 2, No. 6, p. 34.
8. Huelsenbeck, Richard, 1969. "Reflections on leaving America for good." *American Scholar*. Vol. 39, No. 1, p. 80–85.
9. **Taperibá:** See Materia Medica No. 80, p. 210.
10. **Sangre de grado:** See Materia Medica No. 33, p. 192.
11. **Babassu:** *Orbygnia speciosa*, a palm.
12. **Tahuari negro:** *Tabebuia* sp.
13. **Bellaco caspi:** See Materia Medica No. 7, p. 179.
14. **Socoba:** *Bellaco caspi. op. cit.*
15. Churo: Large forest snail.

Chapter 16: Shaman Master

1. Energy Medicine Bibliography:

Master, R. E. L. and Houston, Jean, 1966. *The Varieties of Psychedelic Experience*. New York: Dell. p. 316.

Rørvik, David, 1973. "The theta experience," *Saturday Review: The Sciences*. May, p. 51.

Aaronson, Steve, 1974. "Pictures of an unknown aura." *Saturday Review: The Sciences*. Vol. 14, No. 1, pp. 15–22.

Grossinger, Richard, 1980. *Planet Medicine*. Boulder: Shambhala (especially "Darwinism, Vitalism, New Alchemy, and Parapsychology," pp. 116–131; and "The Spectrum of Life Energy," pp. 372–401).

Calderón, Eduardo; Cowan, Richard; Sharon, Douglas; and Sharon, F. Kaye, 1982. *Eduardo el Curandero: The Words of a Peruvian Healer*. Berkeley: North Atlantic Books.

Coulter, Harris L. *Homoeopathic Science and Modern Medicine: The Physics of Healing with Microdoses*, 1981. Berkeley: North Atlantic Books.

Whitmont, Edward C., 1980. *Psyche and Substance*. Berkeley: North Atlantic Books.

Fulder, Stephen, 1980. *The Root of Being: Ginseng and the Pharmacology of Harmony*. London: Hutchison.

Dossey, Larry, 1982. *Space, Time & Medicine*. Boulder: Shambhala.

Inglis, Brian, 1965. *The Case for Unorthodox Medicine*. New York: G. P. Putnam's Sons.

Thakkur, Chandrashekhar, G., 1974. *Ayurveda: The Indian Art & Science of Medicine*. New York: ASI Publishers.

Grossinger, Richard (editor). "Alchemy: pre-Egyptian Legacy, Millennial Promise," in *The Alchemical Tradition in the Late Twentieth Century*. Berkeley: North Atlantic Books, 1983.

2. Weil, Andrew, 1972. *The Natural Mind*. Boston: Houghton-Mifflin. pp. 171, 184.

3. *Vinca rosea*: Solomon, Joan, 1971. "Chemotherapy of cancer," *The Sciences*. Vol. 11, No. 4, p. 8.

4. Lapachol: Hooker, S. C. et al. Mem. Vol. ed. by L. F. Fiesser,

1936. "The Constitution and Properties of Lapachol." p.38. It is of interest to note that in the U. S. health food and herbal remedy trade in the 1980s shredded bark of *pau d'arco* from Brazil has become a fast moving item, at times unavailable because of the demand.
5. Weil, Andrew, 1972. *op. cit.*
6. Alejandro Zaffaroni in *Wall Street Journal*, June 18, 1973, p. 32.
7. Rumrill, Roger, 1971. "Este hombre derroto al cancer," *Trinchera*, Vol. 2, No. 6, p. 18. Lima, Peru.

Materia Medica

1. Ames, Oaks. 1969. *Economic Annuals and Human Cultures*. Cambridge: Botanical Museum of Harvard University.

Background Sources

Brown, Barbara, B. 1974. *New Mind, New Body: Biofeedback: New Directions for the Mind*. New York: Harper and Row.

Dobkin de Rios, Marlene. 1973. *Visionary Vine*. Prospect Heights: Waveland Press.

1984. *Hallucinogens: Cross-Cultural Perspectives*. Albuquerque: University of New Mexico Press.

Dubos, Rene. 1968. *Man, Medicine and Environment*. New York: New American Library.

Furst, Peter. (ed.) 1972. *Flesh of the Gods: The Ritual Use of Hallucinogens*. New York: Praeger.

Harner, Michael J. (ed,) 1973. *Hallucinogens and Shamanism*. New York: Oxford University Press.

Jonas, Gerald. 1972. *Visceral Learning*. New York: Viking Press.

Leary, Timothy. 1983. *Flash Backs*. Los Angeles: Tarcher.

Masters, R. E. L. and Jean Houston. 1966. *Varieties of Psychedelic Experience*. New York: Delta.

Naranjo, Claudio. 1973. *The Healing Journey: New Approaches to Consciousness*. New York: Pantheon.

Schultes, Richard E. and Albert Hofmann. 1973. *The Botany and Chemistry of Hallucinogens*. Springfield: Charles Thomas.

Steward, Julian H. (ed.) 1948. *Handbook of South American Indians*. Washington, D.C.: Smithsonian Institution, Bureau of American Ethnology. Bulletin #143.

Swain, Tony. (ed.) 1972. *Plants in the Development of Modern Medicine*. Cambridge: Harvard University Press.

Weil, Andrew. 1972. *The Natural Mind*. Boston: Houghton Mifflin.

1983. *Health and Healing*. Boston: Houghton Mifflin.

Index

Index